Female Genital Mutilation

A handbook for professionals
working in health, education,
social care and the police

Dr Sharon Raymond, MBBS MRCGP

Female Genital Mutilation

A handbook for professionals working in health, education, social care and the police

By Dr Sharon Raymond MBBS MRCGP

© Pavilion Publishing and Media Ltd

The author has asserted her rights in accordance with the Copyright, Designs and Patents Act (1988) to be identified as the author of this work.

Published by:
Pavilion Publishing and Media Ltd
Rayford House, School Road,
Hove, BN3 5HX

Tel: 01273 434943
Fax: 01273 227308
Email: info@pavpub.com
Web: www.pavpub.com

Published 2015.

ISBN: 978-1-910366-41-7

Epub: 978-1-910366-54-7

Epdf: 978-1-910366-55-4

Mobi: 978-1-910366-56-1

A catalogue record for this book is available from the British Library.

Author: Dr Sharon Raymond MBBS MRCGP
Production editor: Mike Benge, Pavilion Publishing and Media Ltd
Cover design: Emma Dawe, Pavilion Publishing and Media Ltd
Layout design: Emma Dawe, Pavilion Publishing and Media Ltd
Printing: CMP Digital Print Solutions

For the girls

Contents

About the author

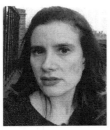 **Dr Sharon Raymond** has worked as a doctor in primary and secondary care, including in prison and army settings, both in the UK and internationally.

She is a medical lead for Care UK primary care out of hours service in North West London and Safeguarding Adults and Children Subject Matter Expert for Care UK, nationally. In addition she works as the Named GP for safeguarding children for Croydon CCG, having previously worked as the Named GP for safeguarding children for Camden CCG. She trains clinicians in level 3 safeguarding children and adults, running the safeguarding adults training in conjunction with the GMC. Dr Raymond's level 3 safeguarding children training with its particular emphasis on the management of FGM has been published on the NHS England pin board as an example of best practice.

Dr. Raymond is a member of the GMC Task and Finish Group on Confidentiality and a Medical Member of the First Tier tribunal Social Entitlement chamber, SSCS.

She has a special interest in FGM and is a member of the NHS England FGM health steering committee, and she has lectured widely to healthcare and allied professionals and written articles for professional journals on FGM.

Introduction

One survivor's experience: the hidden scar

While I had an acute sense of the emotional, psychological and physical implications for survivors of female genital mutilation, it was brought home to me when, on the 23rd May 2014, I heard a survivor's story at first hand. As I listened attentively to her experiences of undergoing female genital mutilation (FGM) as an 11-year-old child in Sierra Leone I fought hard to suppress my tears, as did most other healthcare professionals in the room on that day.

She told how she had been prepared for the day of her coming of age by her mother and grandmother; she would soon become a woman, a member of the Bondo Society, and party to the women's closed sisterhood. In this woman's culture, the practice of FGM had been espoused in order to establish the virginal purity of the girls in her community, with those females not undergoing the procedure at risk of being labelled as promiscuous and dishonourable.

Though her family were poor, she would be showered with gifts and pretty dresses in preparation for this great occasion. She had no idea what awaited her as she celebrated the occasion, dancing excitedly as she was taken blindfolded, like the many other girls with her, to a hut, forcefully pinned down by several women, and without any warning, cut with the same non-sterile implement used on her similarly unsuspecting peers who were all cut on that day. She squealed in agony, so loudly that the beating of the drums in the background could not drown out her persistent cries. Three days later when she went with the other girls to bathe in the river, it was discovered by the village matriarchs that she had been incompletely cut. She was dragged kicking and screaming, this time aware of the fate that awaited her, to undergo the procedure again in order to ensure that it was complete.

She described how, since that time, married life and childbirth have been tarnished by continual physical and emotional pain. Her way of coming to terms with this traumatic experience and its harsh sequelae has been to devote time and energy to campaigning against FGM in the UK. The wounds inflicted by this experience have harmed this survivor both physically and psychologically, and she describes it as a scar that cannot be seen. A hidden scar.

Women and girls should be safeguarded from FGM and survivors of FGM need the right help and support to ensure that any complications are appropriately managed. It is important to bear in mind that a survivor may not be aware that the complications she is experiencing as a direct result of FGM are due to her having undergone this procedure. Indeed, she may not even know that she has undergone FGM, particularly if she underwent the procedure at a very young age, despite suffering from the consequences.

FGM in the UK

Female genital mutilation is illegal in the UK and is a form of abuse against women and girls. The practice confers no health benefits and, as this survivor's experience illustrates, it can lead to significant harm and, in the worst cases, may even be fatal. It may occur in association with other forms of violence against women and girls, such as domestic abuse, forced marriage and honour-based violence.

Tackling FGM is high on the government's agenda. The Home Office published a strategy for tackling violence against women and girls in November 2010, known as the Call to End Violence Against Women and Girls (VAWG) strategy. Action plans are published annually in March, updating the government's work towards the strategy.

All health professionals should have the knowledge and skills to identify when FGM has taken place and be aware of the health implications. Furthermore, healthcare professionals should be able to detect any indicators of risk signalling that FGM may be about to happen.

In its June 2014 report, The Home Affairs Committee on female genital mutilation identified a worrying deficiency in awareness of FGM among professionals, stating as follows:

> 'It is deeply concerning that so many frontline practitioners do not recognise the indicators of when a girl or young woman is at risk, or has undergone FGM, and, even when they do recognise the signs, they do not know how to respond. It is unacceptable that those in a position with the most access to evidence of these crimes do nothing to help the victims and those at risk. The record of referrals by healthcare practitioners and others is extremely poor and a lack of training, awareness or ethical concerns can no longer prevent positive action being taken. To remove one of the obstacles to referring, high-quality training for all professionals, including midwives, GPs, health visitors, practice nurses, teachers, obstetricians and gynaecologists, social workers and teaching assistants, is therefore vital both during education and through continued professional development.'

(Home Affairs Committee, 2014. © Crown copyright. Contains Parliamentary information licensed under the Open Parliament Licence v3.0. To view this license, visit www. nationalarchives.gov.uk/doc/open-government-licence/)

The government has subsequently issued a cross-government declaration highlighting its continued commitment to tackling FGM and forced marriage.

It states:

> '...the Prime Minister and UNICEF hosted the first Girl Summit, aimed at mobilising domestic and international efforts to end female genital mutilation (FGM) and child, early and forced marriage (CEFM) within a generation.
>
> 'The Girl Summit launched a global movement against FGM and CEFM, with over 180 commitments from a range of governments and civil society actors worldwide towards ending the practices, and over 490 pledges for the 'Girl Summit Charter'.
>
> 'In the past year there has been huge progress. Action taken by the UK Government, survivors, voluntary sector partners, and frontline professionals has put preventing and tackling FGM and CEFM firmly on the national agenda. The UK has taken bold action to meet the commitments made at the Summit, including work to safeguard children from harm, strengthen the law, improve the law enforcement response, support frontline professionals, and work with communities.
>
> 'Things are changing. Women and girls are increasingly speaking out, and more and more people are saying no to these practices. Across the UK Government we undertake to build on this momentum and continue to do all we can to protect girls and women and to end FGM and CEFM within a generation.'

(Home Office *et al*, 2015)

The declaration goes on to outline key achievements and next steps, including:

- The Department for International Development's £35 million programme to help the Africa-led movement to end FGM in 17 countries.

- The Home Office has launched a specialist FGM unit and funded a campaign to raise awareness of FGM and 12 community engagement projects.

- HM Inspectorate will conduct a review into honour-based violence, including FGM, to improve police responses.

- The Ministry of Justice has introduced the Serious Crime Act (2015), which has many implications for FGM. For more information, see p31.

- The Department of Health has a £3 million FGM prevention programme underway, and will take the next steps of improving NHS safeguarding systems and working to improve care for the mental health of victims of FGM.

- The Department for Education has funded a £2 million national programme to create a specialised team of skilled social workers with extensive experience of working with those at risk of FGM.

- The Department for Communities and Local Government and the Government Equalities Office have funded 15 community projects to address FGM and forced marriage, as well as establishing community champions against them.

- The Crown Prosecution Service (CPS) has appointed FGM prosecutors for each CPS Area, and have agreed local police/ CPS FGM Protocols with the 43 police force areas, setting out the arrangements for investigation and prosecution of FGM.

(Home Office *et al*, 2015)

To read the whole declaration, which includes more comprehensive details of these achievements and goals, see https://www.gov.uk/government/ publications/declaration-on-uk-government-progress-since-girl-summit-2014 (accessed August 2015).

Healthcare professionals play a key role in supporting patients and managing the complications of FGM, which may be devastating. They also have a duty to protect patients at risk of this harmful practice. This entails ensuring that adults and children are safeguarded from this form of abuse by means of existing child and adult safeguarding mechanisms, policies and procedures. No one single agency can manage the needs of FGM survivors or those at risk of FGM. Therefore the appropriate management of these patients requires good multi-agency working, a recurrent theme identified as lacking in many Serious Case Reviews. FGM has been highlighted as a mandatory competency in the latest intercollegiate guidance document of March 2014 entitled *Safeguarding Children and Young People, Roles and competences for healthcare staff* (RCPCH, 2014)

The duties of healthcare professionals in managing the needs of survivors of FGM and safeguarding patients at risk of FGM, both children and vulnerable adults, have been further formalised by means of UK legislation including The FGM Act (2003), The Prohibition of Female Genital Mutilation (Scotland) Act (2005), The Serious Crime Bill (2015) and The Care Act (2014).

This handbook is geared towards healthcare professionals, including doctors, nurses and health visitors, as well as professionals working alongside healthcare professionals, including social workers, teachers and the police. It aims to outline the background to FGM and to increase professionals' knowledge and skills in identifying and managing those who may be at risk of FGM or who have undergone this practice in line with best practice guidelines and the current legislation. I trust that it will serve to enhance healthcare professionals' understanding and confidence in managing patients who present with FGM and those who may be at risk of this harmful practice.

References

Home Affairs Committee (2014) *Home Affairs Committee – Second Report: Female genital mutilation: the case for a national action plan* [online]. Available at: http://www.publications. parliament.uk/pa/cm201415/cmselect/cmhaff/201/20106.htm#a9 (accessed August 2015).

Home Office (2010-2015) *Call to End Violence Against Women and Girls* [online]. London: Home Office. Available at: https://www.gov.uk/government/publications/call-to-end-violence-against-women-and-girls (accessed August 2015).

Home Office *et al* (2015) Declaration on UK government progress since Girl Summit 2014 [online]. Available at: www.gov.uk/government/publications/declaration-on-uk-government-progress-since-girl-summit-2014 (accessed August 2015).

RCPCH (2014) *Safeguarding Children and Young People: Roles and competences for health care staff, intercollegiate document* [online]. London: Royal College of Paediatrics and Child Health. Available at: http://www.rcn.org.uk/__data/assets/pdf_file/0008/474587/Safeguarding_Children_-_ Roles_and_Competences_for_Healthcare_Staff_02_0....pdf (accessed August 2015)

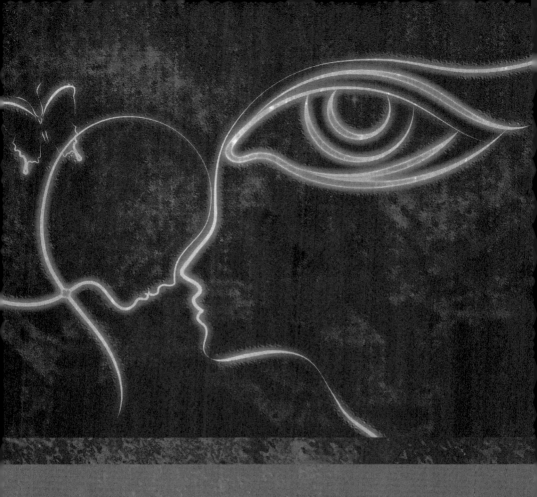

Part one:

An introduction to FGM

Part one: An introduction to FGM

Female genital mutilation is defined by the World Health Organization as comprising all procedures that involve partial or total removal of the external female genitalia, or other injury to the female genital organs for non-medical reasons. For the purpose of the criminal law in England, Wales and Northern Ireland, FGM refers to the partial or total removal or other injury to the labia majora, labia minora or clitoris.

FGM is a practice dating back some 2,000 years to ancient Egypt and, although not explicitly mentioned, is alluded to in the Bible as a practice performed on Egyptian slaves. It is prevalent in 28 African countries, parts of the Middle East and Asia where the practice is deeply embedded (see Figure 1.2 on p19), and due to increasing migration, it is becoming more prevalent in the UK.

Terminology

FGM is also known as female genital cutting and female circumcision. The term 'female genital mutilation' is used in this handbook as it is the term generally applied in professional literature, including clinical guidelines and legislation.

However, it is important for healthcare professionals to ensure that they employ the utmost sensitivity in the terminology they use when communicating with patients, as the term 'mutilation' may carry negative connotations for patients that may impact on their self-esteem. It is likely that most patients would prefer to be referred to as 'survivors' rather than 'mutilated'.

Furthermore, patients may be unfamiliar with the term 'female genital mutilation' and it would be preferable to refer to 'cutting', 'female circumcision', being 'opened' or 'closed' or to use colloquial terms (see Table 1.1) when communicating with patients.

Table 1.1: Traditional and local terms for FGM

Country	Term used for FGM	Language	Meaning
Egypt	Thara	Arabic	Deriving from the Arabic word 'tahar', meaning to clean/purify
	Khitan	Arabic	Circumcision – used for both FGM and male circumcision
	Khifad	Arabic	Deriving from the Arabic word 'khafad' meaning to lower (rarely used in everyday language)
Ethiopia	Megrez	Amharic	Circumcision/cutting
	Absum	Harrari	Name giving ritual
Eritrea	Mekhnishab	Tigregna	Circumcision/cutting
Kenya	Kutairi	Swahili	Circumcision – used for both FGM and male circumcision
	Kutairi was ichana	Swahili	Circumcision of girls
Nigeria	Ibi/Ugwu	Igbo	The act of cutting – used for both FGM and male circumcision
	Sunna	Mandingo	Religious tradition/obligation – for Muslims
Sierra Leone	Sunna	Soussou	Religious tradition/obligation – for Muslims
	Bondo	Temenee/ Mandingo/ Limba	Integral part of initiation rite into adulthood – for non-Muslims
	Bondo/Sonde	Mendee	Integral part of initiation rite into adulthood – for non-Muslims
Somalia	Gudiniin	Somali	Circumcision – used for both FGM and male circumcision
	Halalays	Somali	Deriving from the Arabic word 'halal' i.e. 'sanctioned' – implies purity. Used by northern and Arabic speaking Somalis
	Qodiin	Somali	Stitching/tightening/sewing refers to infibulation (see 'Definition and types' on p11)

Country	Term used for FGM	Language	Meaning
Sudan	Khifad	Arabic	Deriving from the Arabic word 'khafad' meaning to lower (rarely used in everyday language)
	Tahoor	Arabic	Deriving from the Arabic word 'tahar', meaning to clean/purify
Chad – the Ngama	Bagne		Used by Sara Madjingaye
Sara subgroup	Gadja		Adapted from 'ganza' used in the Central African Republic
Guinea-Basau	Fanadu di mindjer	Kriolu	Circumcision of girls
Gambia	Niaka	Mandinka	Literally to 'cut/weed clean'
	Kuyango	Mandinka	Meaning 'the affair' but also the name of the shed built for initiates
	Musolula Karoola	Mandinka	Meaning 'the woman's side'/'that which concerns women'

(Department of Health, 2015)

Female genital mutilation: definition and types

FGM covers all procedures involving the partial or total removal of the external female genitalia or other injury to the female genital organs for non-medical reasons. The practice entails the removal and/or damaging of normal female genital tissue and can interfere with the normal function of the female body.

It confers no health advantages and may lead to short and long-term physical and psychological complications (see 'The complications of FGM' on p14), and in the worst cases can cause the death of a female and/or her child due to complications in pregnancy and/or labour.

The World Health Organization has classified FGM into four main types, all of which are illegal in the UK.

Confidently diagnosing the type of FGM undergone by a patient may pose a challenge for healthcare professionals, and may not be clinically evident at all in some cases, particularly in the case of Type 4 FGM, below.

Type 1 FGM: cliteroidectomy

Type 1 is defined by WHO as the partial or total removal of the clitoris (a small, sensitive and erectile part of the female genitals) or, in very rare cases, only the prepuce (the fold of skin surrounding the clitoris). (WHO, 2014.)

Type 2 FGM: excision

Type 2 is defined by WHO as the partial or total removal of the clitoris and the labia minora, with or without excision of the labia majora (the labia are the 'lips' that surround the vagina) (WHO, 2014).

Type 3 FGM: infibulation

Type 3 FGM is defined by WHO as the narrowing of the vaginal opening through the creation of a covering seal. The seal is formed by cutting and repositioning the inner or outer labia, with or without removal of the clitoris (WHO, 2014).

Type 3 is deemed to protect women and girls from sexual promiscuity and, in certain cultures, the husband and family members ensure that the new bride is cut open in preparation for her wedding night.

Type 4 FGM: other

According to WHO, type 4 constitutes all other harmful procedures to the female genitalia for non-medical purposes e.g. pricking, piercing, incising, scraping and cauterising the genital area. It is important to note that type 4 includes genital piercings (WHO, 2014).

Figure 1.1: Types of FGM

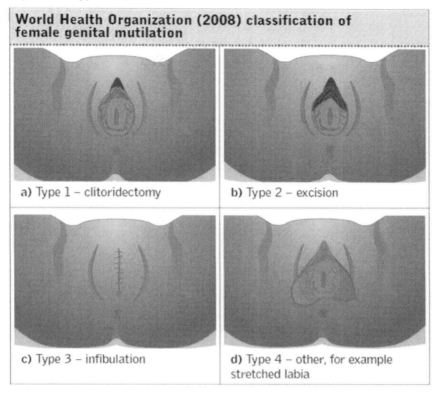

a) Type 1 – clitoridectomy

b) Type 2 – excision

c) Type 3 – infibulation

d) Type 4 – other, for example stretched labia

Women may undergo the procedure after childbirth in order to restore the narrow vaginal opening created by type 3 FGM and widened in childbirth. This is termed reinfibulation and may be performed after each child is born.

How is FGM carried out and by whom?

FGM is thought to be performed on British girls in the UK and abroad (often in the family's country of origin). School-aged girls tend to undergo FGM abroad, often being taken abroad at the start of the school holidays to allow adequate time for recovery before the start of the next term.

FGM is often undertaken by an older female in the community. The role of 'cutter' carries with it prestige and can be financially rewarding. These traditional circumcisers tend to have a pivotal role in other events within communities such as childbirths, and are viewed as respected elders of the community. It is also important to remember that female cutters will themselves have undergone FGM.

The survivor's story in the introduction of this handbook is fairly typical of how FGM is carried out in countries where it has not been medicalised. Often the girl or young woman will be forcibly pinned down by a number of older women. The cutter is unlikely to have any clinical expertise, and will generally not use any anaesthetic, nor perform the procedure under sterile conditions. A variety of implements may be used to perform FGM and the same instrument will tend to be used on more than one girl or woman. These implements may include the following: razors, stones, broken glass and knives.

As in the case of the survivor's story related in the introduction of this book, the woman or girl often is not aware that she is about to be cut. This lack of preparation compounds the ensuing emotional shock and psychological trauma.

Today, however, it has become increasingly common for FGM to be undertaken by medical professionals within clinics, with over 18% of all FGM worldwide being performed by healthcare providers, for example in Egypt, where more than 75% of cases of FGM are performed by medical practitioners.

While this may reduce pain at the time of the procedure, decrease the chance of infection, as well as limit the possibility of some of the physical complications immediately post-procedure, it does not prevent the risk of longer term physical and psychological complications. FGM is an abuse of women and girls leading to harm both physical and psychological, no matter where it is performed or who performs it.

The complications of FGM

Physical complications

FGM may lead to severe physical and psychological complications, which can occur at the time the FGM is performed, soon after, or as late complications. It is common for families and communities to ignore the complications of FGM due to embarrassment, fear of consequences of speaking out against a valued cultural practice and/or lack of awareness of an association between FGM and the complications that may result. Women, girls and communities may not be aware of the complications that result due to FGM being undertaken at a young age, including in particular those complications impacting on intimate relationships, childbirth and the emotional and psychological sequelae.

Healthcare professionals have a central role in identifying a possible link between a range of complications and FGM, including in cases where the woman or girl is unaware that she has undergone the procedure. The World Health Organisation has highlighted that all types of FGM, in particular type 3, can lead to complications in childbirth, including in some cases death of the mother and her child.

Early physical complications include the following:

- Damage to soft tissues, bones and organs due to being forcibly restrained.
- Haemorrhage.
- Extreme pain.
- Infections, both local and systemic, including tetanus, hepatitis B and C, HIV.
- Urinary retention.
- Death.

The late physical complications include the following:

- Complications in pregnancy and delayed second stage of labour, particularly in type 3 FGM, which may lead to the death of mother and child, perinatally. Women and girls who have undergone all types of FGM, even after deinfibulation, are at increased risk in pregnancy and childbirth of the following: caesarian section, perineal trauma (such as third degree tears and episiotomy) and post-partum haemorrhage.
- Obstetric fistulas.
- Infections, including chronic and recurrent vaginal and pelvic infections, urine infections, systemic infections.
- Difficulty passing urine, particularly in type 3 FGM.
- Impaired renal function, including renal failure.
- Menstrual problems, including blockage of menstrual flow in type 3 FGM.
- Gynaecological complications including infertility.
- Dyspareunia and lack of pleasure during sexual intercourse.
- Infibulation cysts, neuromas and keloid scarring locally.

An internet search will return a number of results showing some of the implements used, the procedures and complications of FGM.

Please note that some of these images are graphic and some people may find them disturbing.

The World Health Organization Study Group on Female Genital Mutilation and Obstetric Outcome (WHO, 2006) demonstrated that pregnant women with previous FGM have an increased risk of haemorrhage, perineal trauma, caesarean section and perinatal death.

Box 1.1: A note on medical examinations

The Multi-Agency Practice Guidelines: Female genital mutilation (HM Government, 2014) state:

'Intimate medical examinations to identify or determine FGM presence are not carried out in the NHS. In some cases however, it may be necessary to seek a medical examination for emotional or physical conditions. It may not be advisable to call or visit a medical practitioner from the local community as this may threaten the security of the victim.

The General Medical Council (GMC) have issued guidance on child protection examinations at http://www.gmc-uk.org/guidance/ethical_ guidance/13431.asp. Consent or other legal authorisation is required to carry out any child protection examination, including a psychiatric or psychological assessment. The GMC guidance also outlines the steps to take when consent to examination is not given.

It is mandatory for health professionals to record in their healthcare record if a patient has FGM whenever it is identified in the course of NHS treatment. It is also advisable in all cases where injuries are apparent to encourage the person to have those injuries documented for future reference.

Remember:
Any examination of a child or young person should be in strict accordance with safeguarding children procedures and should [normally] be carried out by a consultant paediatrician, preferably with experience of dealing with cases of FGM.

The GMC has issued ethical guidance on child protection which outlines how to identify risk, considerations around confidentiality and procedures to follow. The guidance can be accessed at: http:// www.gmc-uk.org/guidance.

(HM Government, 2014)

Psychological complications

FGM is perceived by communities as an 'act of love', undertaken for the betterment of a girl's life and to promote her acceptance into society as a chaste and marriageable woman, in accordance with cultural precepts. In the immediate aftermath of FGM, a woman or girl may be profoundly shocked by this practice having been arranged by loving parents and a caring community.

Evidence from survivors has illustrated that FGM is a highly traumatic procedure for women and girls, the memory of which persists for the rest of their lives. Women receiving psychological counselling in the UK have described feeling betrayed by their parents, a sense of incompleteness, regret and anger (Lockhat, 2004).

Severe psychological consequences have increasingly been observed to be associated with FGM and may lead to mental health disorders. Research among practising African communities undertaken by Behrendt and Moritz (2005) showed that women who have had FGM have the same levels of post-traumatic stress disorder (PTSD) as adults who have experienced early childhood abuse, and that most of the women (80%) suffer from affective (mood) or anxiety disorders. The fact that FGM is deeply rooted in the community does not protect a survivor from developing PTSD and other psychiatric disorders.

Psychological complications may include the following:

- Psychosexual problems, including sexual dysfunction and low libido.
- Depression, including possible self-harm and substance misuse.
- Anxiety.
- PTSD – flashbacks may be triggered by pregnancy and childbirth.

Psychological/mental health support is a key element in best managing FGM, along with appropriate management of physical symptoms and complications.

Motives for performing FGM

The exact origin of FGM is not known and a varied range of motives have been identified for performing FGM within practising communities, but whatever the motives, it tends to represent a deeply rooted custom and tradition. In some countries, FGM may be used as a political tool and a means of exerting control.

For those who practice it, FGM is thought to constitute a rite of passage for a girl into womanhood and is therefore part of being a woman. It is perceived as integral to 'cleansing' and preserving a girl's purity and chastity, and ensuring her acceptance within her community, and therefore guarantees that she is marriageable. Conversely, a girl or woman who has not had FGM because she has refused to undergo it or who may have reported it or spoken out against the practice, may be shunned by her family and community with potentially far-reaching socio-economic consequences. Furthermore, it is thought to preserve the wider family's honour and ensure that they are accepted within their society, and hence a daughter's rejection of FGM may impact on a whole family's honour within their community.

FGM therefore tends to be carried out by families with the support and encouragement of their communities as an act of love, with the intention of performing what is held by them to be a beneficial practice undertaken in her best interests. A girl or young woman who does not undergo FGM may be regarded as unmarriageable, or be ostracised by her community for eschewing the practice.

As a result of this, a girl or woman may be reluctant to come forward and report that she has undergone FGM, or that she is at risk of FGM being carried out, due to a fear of hurting her loved ones.

Some communities claim that there is a religious justification for FGM, however there is no basis for the practising of FGM in any religious text. FGM predates Christianity, Islam and Judaism, and no religious text promotes nor justifies it. In 2006, Muslim clerics at an international conference on FGM in Egypt declared that FGM is not Islamic, and the London Central Mosque has stated that FGM entails harming oneself or others, which is forbidden within Islam.

Some communities believe that FGM makes childbirth safer for a baby. It is also thought that FGM protects the family from evil spirits and misfortune.

The age at which FGM is carried out varies greatly between practising communities. It may be performed from the newborn period to adolescence, or just before marriage, as well as during pregnancy and after childbirth. In the latter case, FGM may be carried on multiple occasions after the birth of each child. While FGM may be performed at any age, the peak prevalence appears to be five to eight years of age and this age range is therefore considered high risk.

Bearing in mind that FGM is illegal, many patients may not even be aware that they have undergone the procedure, particularly if it has been carried out at a very young age. Healthcare professionals may therefore be in a position to join the dots and identify that the symptoms a patient has presented with may in fact be complications due to FGM.

Demographics and prevalence

FGM is prevalent in 28 African countries, parts of the Middle East and Asia. The practice of FGM is focused in a cluster of countries from the Atlantic coast to the Horn of Africa.

In order to obtain an indication of the prevalence of FGM in Liberia, women and girls were asked whether they were members of the Sande society, as initiation into this society entails undergoing FGM. FGM has also been documented in communities in:

- India
- Indonesia
- Israel
- Malaysia
- Oman
- Pakistan
- Palestinian Territories
- United Arab Emirates

Figure 1.2: Geographical prevalence of FGM

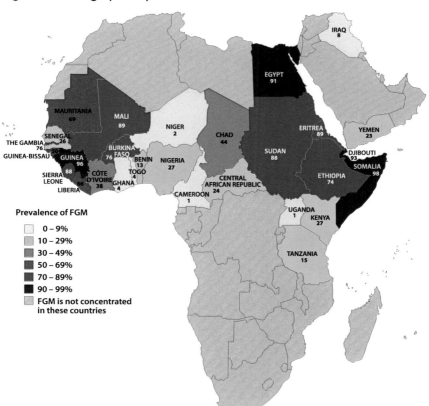

Prevalence of FGM

- 0 – 9%
- 10 – 29%
- 30 – 49%
- 50 – 69%
- 70 – 89%
- 90 – 99%
- FGM is not concentrated in these countries

(Department of Health, 2015) Source: UNICEF global databases, 2014, based on DHS, MICS and other nationally representative surveys, 2004-2013. Available at: http://www.data.unicef.org/child-protection/fgmc

The World Health Organization has estimated that between 100 and 140 million girls and women worldwide have undergone FGM and approximately three million girls experience FGM every year in Africa.

The Department of Health is collecting data regarding UK figures for FGM, known as the FGM Prevalence Dataset, with mandatory data gathering currently being undertaken by acute trusts. Primary care is due to commence FGM data collection by October 2015 as guided by the HSCIC.

A recent study by Macfarlane and Dorkenoo (2014) estimated prevalence figures for FGM in England and Wales, and calculated that about 137,000 women and girls in England and Wales are survivors of FGM. They estimated that there are approximately 103,000 women aged 15-49 and 24,000 women aged 50 and over who have migrated to England and Wales having undergone FGM, and approximately 10,000 girls aged under 15 who have migrated to England and Wales likely to have undergone FGM. The study further estimated that about 60,000 girls up to the age of 14 years were born in England and Wales to mothers who had undergone FGM.

Due to population growth and immigration from practising countries since 2001, FGM may in fact be significantly more prevalent than these estimated figures.

It is worth noting that there may be certain geographical foci of cases of FGM within the UK, with more occurring in those areas of the UK with larger communities from the practising countries – found by the aforementioned study to be London, Cardiff, Manchester, Sheffield, Northampton, Birmingham, Oxford, Crawley, Reading, Slough and Milton Keynes. However, FGM may be undertaken within families of mixed ethnicities and a woman from a non-practising community whose partner is from a practising community may undergo FGM, along with their daughter(s).

At present, much of the data on FGM in the UK is based on estimated figures.

The FGM Enhanced Dataset: collecting the figures

The FGM Enhanced Information Standard mandates that all clinicians record in the medical records when a patient with FGM is identified, and what type it is. The Department of Health has led a programme of work aimed at improving the management of FGM and those at risk of FGM within the NHS. The data on FGM collated for the FGM Prevalence Dataset will guide the ongoing development and goals of the Department of Health FGM Prevention Programme. The Health and Social Care Information Centre (HSCIC) works alongside the Department of Health to manage and publish the data submitted.

Whenever FGM is identified, not just the first time, and however it has been identified, whether through clinical examination or self-reported by a woman or girl, once recorded in the clinical notes it must be submitted to the data collection.

The full dataset includes: patient demographic data, specific FGM information, referral and treatment information. The FGM Datasets use the World Health Organization's (WHO) definitions for the four types of FGM (see p12).

One of the aims of the FGM Enhanced Dataset, which is to be facilitated by the mandatory reporting of FGM by acute trusts, mental health trusts and primary care, is to collate more precise figures in order to best manage the needs of those who have undergone FGM and to safeguard those who may be at risk of this practice.

Collection and submission of the new dataset became mandatory for all acute trusts from 1 June 2015, and all GPs and mental health trusts from 1 October 2015. Mental health trusts and GPs within areas identified by the Prevalence Dataset as having a prevalence of FGM should forward data from June 2015.

Organisations must submit data quarterly before the extract for the report being taken. Hence the deadline, for example, for the quarter of April-June is the last day of July.

The actions that need to be taken are as follows:

- On receipt of FGM information:
  - a newborn's healthcare record needs updating
  - a mother's healthcare record needs updating.
- When referring a woman/girl with FGM to an applicable clinical setting, include FGM information.
- When applicable, update the Personal Child Health Record (Red Book).
- When there is a family history of FGM, update any sisters' healthcare records.

(HSCIC, 2014)

All data for the FGM Enhanced Dataset is submitted via the HSCIC Clinical Audit Platform http://www.hscic.gov.uk/clinicalauditplatform (CAP). Data can be submitted directly into CAP or via CSV file upload. The CSV specification can be found within the Excel dataset file.

Data could be computer generated if so chosen, or determined locally between organisations and suppliers. This would require the relevant fields to be created in those existing systems, to support the collection of the relevant dataset items, then reported on/extracted appropriately, before being mapped to the CAP upload file to ensure that the collection tool is updated accordingly.

GPs, acute and mental health trusts in England can register to participate by completing a User Registration Form to be found on the HSCIC website. Users can access CAP at: https://clinicalaudit.hscic.gov.uk/fgm

In the period September 2014 to January 2015, the HSCIC reported that over 2,600 patients were treated in the NHS for whom it was newly identified that they have undergone FGM.

For the FGM Enhanced Dataset, the HSCIC is publishing quarterly reports based on extractions from the data collection system. The first report was based on the April – June 2015 quarter.

For the FGM Prevalence Dataset, the HSCIC published monthly reports based on the monthly returns. The first report was published on 16 October 2014, based on the first month of mandated collection, the September 2014 return. The final report was published on 30 April 2015, based on the March 2015 return.

There are some challenges in collating the data. First, it is not automatically extracted from patient records held on the various computer systems used within the NHS and needs to be extracted manually. Second, the Enhanced Dataset mandates the submission of patient names, which may be a barrier in patients agreeing to the submission of their data.

Patient consent relies on ministerial direction, as long as there is fair processing of the data i.e. a patient needs to be informed about what is happening with their data, and if they would like to object to this they can do so by notifying HSCIC. Once the objection is received at the HSCIC an automatic stop processing notice will be issued. The FGM directions go further than usual, in that normally an assessment of the distress caused by collecting the data is made before any further action is taken. The FGM direction ensures that, on submission of an objection to use of a patient's data, an automatic stop process is applied to stop patient data being processed.

Additional patient-identifiable data, including surname, forename and date of birth, are required to confirm the NHS number submitted. Once this has been confirmed and analysis completed, patient-identifiable data is deleted before the publication of official statistics. The collation of FGM data is at patient level in order to ensure that valid data is obtained and to prevent double counting of patients.

For further information, refer to www.hscic.gov.uk/fgm, or for specific queries contact the Health and Social Care Information Centre's Contact Centre on 03003035678 or email enquiries@hscic.gov.uk.

References

Behrendt A & Moritz S (2005) Post traumatic stress disorder and memory problems after female genital mutilation. *American Journal of Psychiatry* **162** 1000–1002.

Department of Health (2015) *FGM Risk and Safeguarding: Guidance for professionals* [online]. London: DoH. Available at: https://www.gov.uk/government/uploads/system/uploads/attachment_data/file/418564/2903800_DH_FGM_Accessible_v0.1.pdf (accessed August 2015).

HSCIC (2014) FGM Enhanced Dataset Implementation Summary for GP Practices [online]. Available at: www.hscic.gov.uk/media/16755/FGM-Enhanced-Dataset-Implementation-Summary-for-GP-Practices/pdf/FGM_Enhanced_Dataset_Implementation_Guidance_Summary_for_GPs_FINAL.pdf (accessed September 2015).

HM Government (2014) *Multi-Agency Practice Guidelines: Female genital mutilation* [online]. London: HM Government. Available at: https://www.gov.uk/government/uploads/system/uploads/attachment_data/file/380125/MultiAgencyPracticeGuidelinesNov14.pdf (accessed August 2015).

Lockhat H (2004) *Female Genital Mutilation: Treating the tears*. London: Middlesex University Press.

Macfarlane A & Dorkenoo E (2014) *Female Genital Mutilation in England and Wales: Updated statistical estimates of the numbers of affected women living in England and Wales and girls at risk* [online]. London: City University London. Available at: http://www.equalitynow.org/sites/default/files/FGM%20EN%20City%20Estimates.pdf (accessed August 2015).

WHO (2006) Female genital mutilation and obstetric outcome: WHO collaborative prospective study in six African countries. *Lancet* **367** (9525) 1835-1841.

WHO (2014) *Female genital mutilation* [online. Available at: www.who.int/mediacentre/factsheets/fs241/en/ (accessed September 2015).

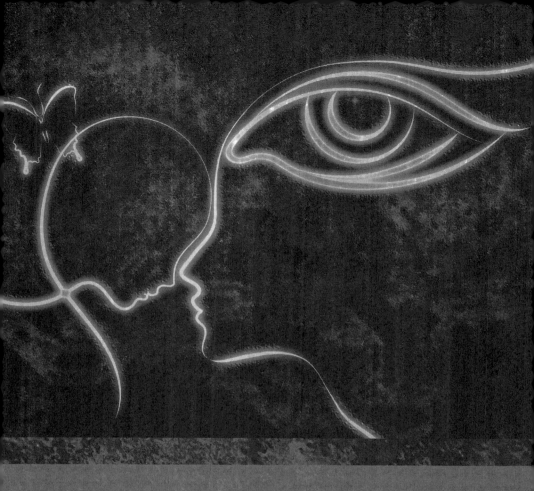

Part two:

FGM and the law

Part two: FGM and the law

The law abroad

FGM is internationally acknowledged to be a contravention of an individual's human rights. It represents a serious form of discrimination against women and girls and contravenes one's right to health, security, personal integrity, the right to be free from torture, cruel, inhumane and degrading abuse, and the right to life when FGM leads to death.

FGM also contravenes The Human Rights Act (1998) and the European Convention on Human Rights, particularly Article 3: that no one will be 'subjected to torture or to inhuman or degrading treatment or punishment'. The UN's Declaration of the Rights of the Child states:

> *'All children shall enjoy special protection, and shall be given opportunities and facilities, by law and by other means, to enable them to develop physically, mentally, morally, spiritually and socially in a healthy and normal manner and in conditions of freedom and dignity.'*

(UN, 1959)

The declaration became the basis of the Convention of the Rights of the Child, which came into force on 2nd September 1990. The convention, ratified by the UK, establishes that anyone under 18 years has the right to be protected from activities or events that may harm them, and that they require the necessary safeguards, including legal protection.

It is important to note that despite international and national legislation against FGM, including in many of the countries that FGM is practised, FGM continues, sometimes in flagrant disregard of legislation put in place in countries whose regimes may tacitly support it. The practice of FGM was outlawed in Egypt in 2008, for example, yet it still has one of the highest rates of prevalence worldwide, and in 2013 a 13-year-old girl died in Egypt following FGM performed by a doctor at a clinic in Aga. Although the doctor was initially acquitted, he was eventually convicted of manslaughter following an appeal. The child's father was given a three-month suspended sentence. This was the first time that a prosecution in relation to FGM had come to trial in Egypt.

FGM is illegal in the following countries where its practice has been prevalent:

- Benin
- Central African Republic

- Chad
- Djibouti
- Egypt
- Eritrea
- Ethiopia
- Ghana
- Guinea
- Ivory Coast
- Kenya
- Niger
- Nigeria
- Senegal
- Tanzania
- Togo
- Uganda

UK Legislation

FGM is illegal in the UK, however there have been no successful convictions to date. In 2014, a doctor working at the Whittington Hospital, London, became the first person in the UK to be prosecuted in relation to FGM however he was acquitted of the offence. In the UK there have only been a handful of reports of FGM to the police – between 2010 and 2013 the Metropolitan Police recorded just 20 referrals of an FGM crime. The Home Affairs Committee on FGM noted in 2014 that the CPS received its first referral from the police in 2010 and had examined 14 cases up to 2014. In France there have been over 100 convictions, although some of these convictions arose from connected cases.

The Home Affairs Committee on FGM in 2014 highlighted that the small number of investigations can be attributed to the following:

'... a reliance on victims or witnesses to report to the police, which they are unlikely to do, and the failure of health, education and social care professionals to refer cases to the police where they suspect FGM to have taken place.'

(Parliament.uk, 2014)

There has been specific legislation in the UK against FGM since the Prohibition of Female Circumcision Act (1985). The Female Genital Mutilation Act (2003) repealed, revised and re-enacted the 1985 legislation, establishing the maximum penalty for this criminal offence as 14 years in prison. Furthermore, the 2003 Act made it a crime for UK nationals or permanent UK residents to perform FGM abroad and to make a UK national or permanent UK resident have FGM. It came into force on 3 March 2004 and applies to England, Northern Ireland and Wales.

Following the introduction of the act, it became illegal to 'excise, infibulate or otherwise mutilate the whole or any part of a female's labia majora, labia minora or clitoris' (HM Government, 2014b), unless performed by a medical practitioner for necessary reasons (section 1(2) and (3)).

Except in these circumstances it is an offence in England, Wales and Northern Ireland to:

■ perform FGM (section 1)

■ assist someone to perform FGM on herself (section 2)

■ assist a non-UK person to perform FGM outside the country on a UK national or UK resident (section 3).

(HM Government, 2014b)

Where FGM takes place in these countries of the UK, issues of nationality or residence status are irrelevant.

The act makes it illegal for a UK national or permanent resident to perform FGM abroad (sections 1 and 4), assist a girl to perform it on herself abroad (sections 2 and 4), or to assist a non-UK person to perform it abroad on a UK national or UK resident (sections 3 and 4). The exceptions for medical professionals performing necessary surgeries also apply to these extra-territorial offences (section 1(4).

The maximum penalty for committing an offence under the act is 14 years imprisonment, a fine, or both.

In Scotland, the Prohibition of Female Genital Mutilation Act (2005), which came into force on 1st September 2005, repealed, revised and re-enacted the 1985 Prohibition of Female Circumcision Act (1985), establishing the maximum prison sentence for FGM at 14 years and making it an offence for UK nationals or permanent UK residents to perform FGM abroad and make a UK national or UK permanent resident have FGM abroad.

> ### Box 2.1: A note on the Health Passport: statement opposing female genital mutilation
>
> In 2014, the government published *A Statement Opposing Female Genital Mutilation*, a leaflet commonly referred to as the Health Passport (HM Government, 2014a).
>
> According to the Department of Health: 'This pocket-sized document sets out the law and the potential criminal penalties that can be used against those allowing FGM to take place. It is designed to be discreetly carried in a purse, wallet or passport.
>
> It can be used by families who have immigrated to the UK and do not want their children to undergo FGM, but still feel pressurised by cultural and social expectations when visiting family and friends abroad. It has been supported and signed by Home Office Ministers, the Department of Health, the Ministry of Justice, the Department for Education and the Director of Public Prosecutions (DPP). In Holland, a similar document is used to support families and has constituted a powerful instrument in establishing that FGM is unacceptable.
>
> Organisations should strive to offer this leaflet to patients routinely when discussing FGM. Copies can be obtained from the Department of Health order line: https://www.orderline.dh.gov.uk.'
>
> (Department of Health, 2015a)

Challenges posed by the legislation

Vaginal piercings and the law

Vaginal piercings constitute type 4 FGM and are therefore illegal as outlined in the FGM Act (2003). Regarding other legislation pertaining to genital piercing, while the Tattooing of Minors Act (1969) sets a statutory minimum age for permanent tattooing of 18 years, there is no statutory minimum age for any type of skin piercing. In some areas of London, local authorities establish a minimum age for skin piercing either banning piercing under the age of 18 or 16, banning all genital or nipple piercing, permitting piercing with parental consent or allowing piercing other than genital piercing over the ages of 16 or 18 years. The law does, however, permit under 18 year olds to consent to cosmetic body piercing provided individuals are mature enough. The Sexual Offences Act (1956) establishes that under 16 year olds cannot consent to intimate sexual contact under any circumstances, hence, piercing of nipples and genitalia may be deemed to be sexual assault. Cases of genital piercing of females under 18 years of age referred to the police will be evaluated on the basis of individual facts and merits, and whether FGM type 4 has been committed will depend on the evidence obtained.

(Public Health England *et al*, 2013.)

Female genital cosmetic surgery and the law

The FGM Act (2003) does not incorporate any explicit exemption for female genital cosmetic surgery. The Home Affairs Select Committee described the laws relating to female genital cosmetic surgery as ambiguous, stating that:

> *'Female genital cosmetic surgery (FGCS) is an increasingly popular form of surgery. For example, there has been a fivefold increase in the number of labiaplasty procedures – the most common form of FGCS – in the last 10 years. However, FORWARD told us such procedures are often very similar to Type 1 and Type 2 FGM, and can result in comparable health complications such as reduced sensation, infection and bleeding, and wound dehiscence. FGCS is mainly performed in the private sector, and so is not subject to the same level of regulation or monitoring as in the NHS. Both ACPO and the Metropolitan Police argued that at present there is a perceived "double standard" whereby there is a focus on practising black and ethnic minority communities, whilst in the wider community the "designer vagina" private medical industry is flourishing.*
>
> *Furthermore, section 1 of the 2003 Act allows for "a surgical operation on a girl which is necessary for her physical or mental health", which the Mayor of London's Harmful Practices Taskforce argued creates a loophole that potentially allows medical practitioners in the private cosmetic industry to conduct FGM with impunity. FORWARD pointed to a recent position paper by the Royal College of Obstetricians and Gynaecologists and the British Society for Paediatric and Adolescent Gynaecology, which recommended that FGCS should not be carried out on girls under the age of 18.'*

(Home Affairs Committee, 2014. Contains Parliamentary information licensed under the Open Parliament Licence v3.0.)

The Serious Crime Act (2015)

The Serious Crime Act (2015)[1] is new legislation to tackle FGM that will:

- Extend the extra-territorial reach of the offences in the Female Genital Mutilation Act (2003) and Prevention of Female Genital Mutilation (Scotland) Act (2005) to refer to habitual residents in the UK as well as permanent UK residents. This part of The Serious Crime Act (2015) will confer the protection of the law on those females who are not permanent UK residents and are at risk of undergoing FGM outside of the UK. (See Box 2.2: A note on immigration status.)

- Introduce a new offence of failure to protect a girl from FGM. In the cases of girls under 16, each individual responsible for the girl when the FGM was performed will be liable under this legislation, with the maximum penalty being seven years imprisonment.

1 For the full legislation, see http://www.legislation.gov.uk/ukpga/2015/9/pdfs/ukpga_20150009_en.pdf

Being 'responsible' for a girl is defined as having parental responsibility and frequent contact with the girl or, in the case of young women aged 18 or over, they will have taken on responsibility for caring for the young woman in what is termed 'the manner of a parent' e.g. family members hosting the individual during holidays.

- Confer lifelong anonymity to those who have undergone FGM.
- Introduce specific civil orders (FGM protection orders) to protect those at risk of FGM.
- Place a mandatory duty on those employed in regulated professions, including teachers, healthcare professionals and social workers, to report to the police when FGM has been performed on a female aged under 18 years. This duty will likely come into force by the end of 2015.

The Serious Crime Act (2015) states that this report:

- *'is to be made to the chief officer of police for the area in which the girl resides*
- *must identify the girl and explain why the notification is made*
- *must be made before the end of one month from the time when the person making the notification first discovers that an act of female genital mutilation appears to have been carried out on the girl*
- *may be made orally or in writing'*

(Serious Crime Act (2015) © Crown Copyright 2015)

According to the Ministry of Justice and the Home Office guidance:

'The duty applies where the professional either:

- *is informed by the girl that an act of FGM has been carried out on her*
- *observes physical signs which appear to show an act of FGM has been carried out and has no reason to believe that the act was necessary for the girl's physical or mental health or for purposes connected with labour or birth.*

The duty does not apply where a professional has reason to believe that another individual working in the same profession has previously made a report to the police in connection with the same act of FGM. For these purposes, professionals regulated by a body which belongs to the Professional Standards Authority are considered as belonging to the same profession.'

This mandatory duty to report FGM in girls under 18 and young women came into force on 1st October 2015. The reporting process is being clarified but is likely to impact on existing guidance regarding referral of suspected and actual cases of FGM cited in the Department of Health documents *Female Genital Mutilation Risk and Safeguarding: Guidance for professionals* (Department of Health, 2015b) and the *Multi-Agency Practice Guidelines: Female Genital Mutilation* (HM Government, 2014b) (see Box 2.2), as well as other national and local referral pathways that have been devised, bearing in mind that a report directly to the police rather than via social care is stipulated.

Box 2.2: A note on immigration status

The *Multi Agency Practice Guidelines: Female genital mutilation* state:

'If the girl or woman is from overseas, fleeing potential FGM and applying to remain in the UK as a refugee is a complicated process and may require professional immigration advice (see https://www.gov.uk/ browse/visas-immigration/asylum for more information about the asylum application process).

Many individuals, especially women, may be extremely frightened by contact with any statutory agency, as they may have been told that the authorities will deport them and/or take their parents or children from them.

Professionals need to be extremely sensitive to these fears when dealing with a victim or potential victim from overseas, even if they have indefinite leave to remain (ILR) or a right of abode, as they may not be aware of their true immigration position. These circumstances make them particularly vulnerable.

If it is discovered that they are in breach of immigration rules (for example, if they have overstayed their visa), remember that they may also require medical treatment, or be the victim of a crime and be traumatised as a result. Guidelines on NHS treatment for overseas visitors can be found at https://www.gov.uk/government/publications/ guidance-on-overseas-visitors-hospital-charging-regulations

Do not allow any investigation of their immigration status to impede police enquiries into an offence that may have been committed against the victim or their children. UK Border Agency officials and police officers may choose to establish an agreement or protocol about how any two simultaneous investigations may work.'

(HM Government, 2014b)

Box 2.3: The Serious Crime Bill

The following is the Royal College of Nursing's (RCN) written evidence (published in January 2015) to the Serious Crime Bill Public Bill Committee outlining the RCN's position with respect to FGM and health professionals and the legal structures that the Serious Crime Act (2015) introduces. The original can be found at: http://www.publications.parliament.uk/pa/cm201415/cmpublic/seriouscrime/memo/sc04.htm

Serious Crime Bill

Written evidence submitted by the Royal College of Nursing (RCN) (SC 04).

1.0 With a membership of more than 420,000 registered nurses, midwives, health visitors, nursing students, health care assistants and nurse cadets, the Royal College of Nursing (RCN) is the voice of nursing across the UK and the largest professional union of nursing staff in the world. RCN members work in a variety of hospital and community settings in the NHS and the independent sector. The RCN promotes patient and nursing interests on a wide range of issues by working closely with the UK Governments, the UK Parliaments and other national and European political institutions, trade unions, professional bodies and voluntary organisations.

1.2 The RCN welcomes the efforts made by the Government to legislate for tackling Female Genital Mutilation (FGM) within the Serious Crime Bill. This briefing sets out the RCN's position regarding FGM and health professionals in regards to the legal structures.

2.0 Intercollegiate report

2.1 In November 2013, the RCN, as part of a unique coalition of royal colleges, trade unions and third sector organisations, published 'Tackling FGM in the UK: Intercollegiate recommendations for identifying, recording and reporting' [1]. This ground-breaking report and collaboration recognises that implementing a comprehensive multi-agency action plan is urgently required to ensure that young girls at risk of undergoing FGM are protected by the existing UK legal framework. The joint report from the Intercollegiate Group sets out nine recommendations aimed at health and social care professionals, who are key to bringing about the changes needed to help eradicate FGM.

2.2 Intercollegiate recommendations for tackling FGM in the UK

1. Treat it as child abuse.
2. Document and collect information.
3. Share that information systematically.
4. Empower frontline professionals.
5. Identify girls at risk and refer them as part of child safeguarding obligations.
6. Report cases of FGM.
7. Hold frontline professionals to account.
8. Empower and support affected girls and young women (both those at risk and survivors).
9. Implement awareness campaign.

2.3 Since the publication of the Intercollegiate report, tackling FGM has quickly become a Government priority, and the RCN very much welcomes the heightened awareness of FGM among parliamentarians, the media and the public.

2.4 The Department of Health has made significant steps to tackle FGM from a health care perspective and rightly recognises that health care professionals are crucial to tackling FGM. As set out in the Intercollegiate report, the RCN encourages a multi-agency approach to the implementation of the measures regarding FGM set out in this Bill. It is imperative that information is shared across health, local authorities, schools and the police to ensure the implementation of comprehensive and integrated strategies for tackling FGM.

2.5 The measures set out in this Bill to amend the current legal framework are very much welcome. However, the RCN is mindful that to ensure their success, appropriate training and education of professionals across health and other agencies is essential. It is crucially important that health professionals are comfortable working with survivors/victims of FGM and are aware of the legal structures in place which are there to benefit women and girls who may have been abused or are at risk of FGM. This will also enhance professional understanding and awareness, as well as wider public awareness of the legal parameters that protect victims/survivors and those at risk of FGM. Much work has been done this year to raise awareness of FGM and this effort must continue.

3.0 Clause 68: Anonymity for victims

3.1 The introduction of anonymity for victims of FGM is a welcome step. It is important, however, that the complexities of FGM are sufficiently considered, in comparison to victims of other crimes. For example, anonymity for victims of FGM might result in children, who have been subjected to FGM, being moved away from their families and communities.

3.2 The RCN is mindful that guidance following this legislation should be explicit in signposting survivors/victims of FGM to relevant support services and ensuring that there is sufficient resourcing of appropriate psychological support. FGM causes death, disability, physical and psychological harm for millions of women every year. The Intercollegiate group found that there is strong evidence of a correlation between FGM and psychiatric disorders, with young girls and women presenting with psychological distress and post-traumatic stress disorder.

3.3 The RCN has continually highlighted concern regarding the loss of services and nursing and midwifery posts in settings which would care for girls and women who require care and support. In August 2014, there were nearly 4,000 nursing mental health posts less than in 2010 [2], an extremely worrying decrease which has negatively affected services, particularly in the community. The RCN's recent Frontline First report highlighted these cuts in stark detail; 'Turning back the clock' [3] reveals that the loss of these vital services means many people experiencing symptoms of mental illness are having to wait extraordinary lengths of time to be treated and cared for.

4.0 Clause 69: Offence for failing to protect

The current law does not see FGM as a criminal dereliction of parents'/guardians' duty to protect their children. The RCN strongly welcomes measures within this Bill to make it a criminal offence for parents' and guardians' who fail to protect girls from FGM. To ensure that parents and guardians understand these new laws, it is important that nurses and midwives working with young families are fully aware of the legal framework. In a wider public health role for nurses and midwives working in these settings, it may be appropriate, should a child be identified as at risk, to inform parents and guardians of the legal ramifications of their actions. This multi-agency approach will encourage further sharing of information and increase levels of reporting and consequentially, prosecutions.

5.0 Clause 70: Protection orders

5.1 A key barrier to achieving a successful prosecution for FGM offences relates to the low levels of reporting of the crime of FGM. The existing laws rely on victims of FGM to report the abuse to the police, despite the majority of victims of FGM being under the age of 10 with some under the age of 5, which is why these new measures are essential.

5.2 The Government recently consulted on the proposal to introduce protection orders, a specific civil law, which could provide an additional tool to prevent and help eliminate FGM, which complements existing criminal law. The proposals suggest that a professional authorised by the courts could make an application for a protection order. For this reason, it is imperative that health professionals are fully engaged and consulted without throughout the process, and in subsequent guidance.

5.3 As part of the Intercollegiate Group, the RCN responded to the Ministry of Justice consultation on its proposal for protection orders. The RCN supports this specific legal measure which will strengthen the case for prosecution, and more importantly, it offers protection to at risk girls and young women. It is appropriate that provisions to protect girls from FGM are placed in statute so that a more comprehensive approach is taken to safeguard these girls. The RCN is encouraged by the protection orders for a number of reasons; they will help to further clarify the role of health care professionals in preventing FGM and they complement the Department of Health's and Home Office's initiatives on the mandatory recording and reporting of all FGM.

5.4 In particular, the RCN is supportive of a range of reporting options being available to victims of FGM; should FGM be prevented, girls may prefer the civil enforcement route over the criminal one. However, to further strengthen the law the RCN believes it is necessary to place a limit on the number of civil breaches before criminal sanctions are imposed.

6.0 Mandatory reporting

6.1 The RCN welcomes steps towards the introduction of mandatory reporting of FGM by health care professionals and will be responding to the current Home Office consultation on this issue in due course.

6.2 At present, it is mandatory to record cases of FGM to safeguarding, to ensure that relevant authorities are informed. The mandatory reporting of FGM to authorities, or potentially the police, will alter the landscape of this issue for health care professionals. The RCN supports efforts to introduce mandatory reporting, which will increase information about the prevalence of FGM; this is an important component which will assist health care professionals, local authorities and the police to prevent and prosecute cases of FGM. These steps send a clear signal that FGM must be treated as a crime and as child abuse. For mandatory reporting to be successful, however, it is crucial that health professionals are sufficiently educated and trained in both identifying FGM and working across agencies to record and report the crime. The RCN believes further efforts should be made by the Department of Health and across Government to encourage this.

6.3 A large number of health care professionals, much like the public, are unaware of the nature of this crime, and how to deal with it effectively. It is imperative that all health care professionals are educated and trained to know that FGM is a crime, and know what to do when they have concerns when a girl or woman is at risk.

6.4 In light of recent developments in this area, the RCN will be publishing updated resource for nurses and midwives early 2015.'

January 2015

[1] http://www.rcn.org.uk/__data/assets/pdf_file/0004/547996/Tackling_FGM_in_the_UK_Intercollegiate_recommendations_for_identifying,_recording_and_reporting.pdf
[2] HSCIC workforce statistics August 2014
[3] http://www.rcn.org.uk/__data/assets/pdf_file/0004/600628/004772.pdf

(Parliament.uk, 2015. © Parliamentary copyright. Contains public sector information licensed under the Open Government License v3.0. To view this document, visit www.nationalarchives.gov.uk/doc/open-governement-licence/)

References

Department of Health (2015a) *Commissioning Services to Support Women and Girls with Female Genital Mutilation*. London: DoH.

Department of Health (2015) *Female Genital Mutilation Risk and Safeguarding: Guidance for Professionals* [online]. London: DoH. Available at: https://www.gov.uk/government/uploads/system/uploads/attachment_data/file/418564/2903800_DH_FGM_Accessible_v0.1.pdf (accessed August 2015).

HM Government (2014a) *A Statement Opposing Female Genital Mutilation* [online]. London: HM Government. Available at: https://www.gov.uk/government/uploads/system/uploads/attachment_data/file/378132/FGMstatementNov14.pdf (accessed August 2015).

HM Government (2014b) *Multi-Agency Practice Guidelines: Female genital mutilation* [online]. London: HM Government. Available at: https://www.gov.uk/government/uploads/system/uploads/attachment_data/file/380125/MultiAgencyPracticeGuidelinesNov14.pdf (accessed August 2015).

Home Affairs Committee (2014) *Female Genital Mutilation: The case for a national action plan* [online]. Available at: http://www.publications.parliament.uk/pa/cm201415/cmselect/cmhaff/201/20102.htm (accessed August 2015).

Parliament.uk (2014) *Female Genital Mutilation: The case for a national action plan* [online]. Available at: www.publications.parliament.uk/pa/cm201415/cmselect/cmhaff/201/20102.htm (accessed August 2015).

Parliament.uk (2015) *Serious Crime Bill* [online]. Available at: www.publications.parliament.uk/pa/cm201415/cmpublic/seriouscrime/memo/sc04.htm (accessed August 2015).

Public Health England *et al* (2013) *Tattooing and Body Piercing Toolkit* [online]. Available at: http://www.cieh.org/assets/0/72/1126/1212/1216/1218/1dd4926c-5601-4da3-a06d-ac205ffde495.pdf (accessed September 2015).

United Nations (1959) *Declaration on the Rights of the Child* [online]. Available at: http://www.unicef.org/malaysia/1959-Declaration-of-the-Rights-of-the-Child.pdf (accessed August 2015).

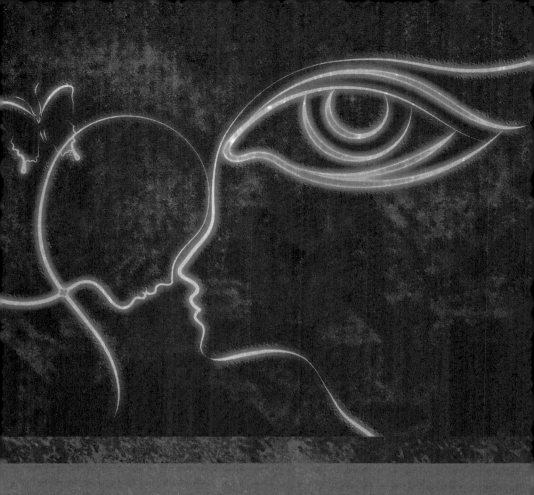

Part three:

Risk assessment, management and safeguarding

Part 3: Risk assessment, management and safeguarding

Risk factors and indicators that FGM is planned

When considering a woman or girl's risk of undergoing FGM, it is important to take into account the following key factors:

- Whether she comes from a practising community (see p19).
- Whether any female member of her family has undergone FGM, particularly her mother and sisters.
- How integrated she and her family are into UK society.
- Has she been removed from Personal, Social and Health Education (PSHE) to restrict her awareness of FGM.

Key indicators that there may be an immediate risk of FGM are:

- a planned visit 'home' to see the family – it is important to bear in mind that families may not travel directly to the country where the FGM may be planned to take place, but rather via another country where FGM is not usually carried out.
- the mention of a special ceremony to mark entry to womanhood.
- an older female relative visiting the UK.
- truancy.
- a plea for help to a trusted adult outside of the community, who may well be a healthcare professional.

It is important to be aware of certain indicators that FGM may have been performed on a woman or girl. A woman or girl may:

- be in obvious discomfort
- have difficulty walking, sitting or standing
- experience pain between the legs

- spend long periods in the toilet due to problems passing urine
- spend long periods away from classes due to bladder or menstrual dysfunction
- experience frequent urinary, menstrual or abdominal symptoms, including chronic pain
- have prolonged or repeated absences from school
- avoid undergoing normal medical examinations, including smear tests and antenatal care
- confide in a professional, disclosing that she has undergone FGM or she may approach a trusted healthcare professional for help without revealing details due to fear of the possible repercussions or embarrassment.

Consultation skills and asking the question

The identification of FGM or a risk of FGM may occur either by means of opportunistic questioning during the course of a consultation prompted by a presenting complaint, or by routine screening. Nationally, women tend to be asked antenatally if they have undergone FGM with a blanket screening approach.

Raising the possibility of FGM with a woman or girl must be handled extremely sensitively in a non-judgemental manner, ensuring a reliance on finely honed clinical skills, as well as a sound knowledge base regarding FGM, including assessment, management, legislation and referral options.

Bearing in mind the complexity and sensitivity of FGM, healthcare professionals should tackle the subject with great care.

The *Multi-Agency Practice Guidelines: Female genital mutilation* state that:

> 'Women often recount feelings of great distress and humiliation due to the responses they receive from professionals when it is revealed that they have been subjected to FGM. They describe looks of horror, inappropriate and insulting questions, and feelings of shame from being made to feel "abnormal". Such negative reactions from professionals are caused by a lack of awareness or understanding of the issue, but can be devastating to a woman who has been subjected to FGM. These stories of negative experiences may reach the communities that practise FGM and could build barriers to the effective care and prevention of FGM, and deter women and girls from seeking treatment or support.

"Sometimes when circumcised women go to the hospital, the nurses call each other to see the circumcised woman. This is an unhappy experience for many women. The nurses ask a lot of questions and they stare."[2]

(HM Government, 2014a)

It would be best practice to ensure that a female professional is available if your patient would prefer this. It is important not to make assumptions and to ensure that a patient is allowed time to talk, and that the healthcare professional conveys the message both verbally and non-verbally that they want to listen. This will facilitate disclosure, which should take place in a confidential setting, respecting the patient's wish either to be alone or with a trusted family member or friend.

Bearing in mind that the practice of FGM is deeply embedded in certain cultures, healthcare professionals must work with patients and their families in a sensitive manner in order to counter any beliefs they might have and to make it clear that FGM is a form of abuse and illegal in the UK, highlighting the range of health complications that may result from it.

Healthcare professionals should take care to be sensitive to patients' race, gender, religion, culture and sexuality and avoid stigmatising patients who have undergone FGM and their communities, bearing in mind safeguarding principles, professional duty of care and the public interest. Fears of being labelled racist should not influence any actions taken to safeguard patients.

Care should be taken to be sensitive to the intimate nature of FGM, and to the fact that patients may have a strong sense of loyalty to parents and their communities, who may have perpetrated FGM as an act of love.

One should take care to be non-judgemental, highlighting that FGM is illegal and leads to complications, but avoid blaming the girl or woman.

The *Multi-Agency Practice Guidelines: Female genital mutilation* state:

'Remember:

- *Individuals may wish to be interviewed by a professional of the same gender.*
- *She may not want to be seen by a professional from her own community.*
- *Alerting the girl's or woman's family to the fact that she is disclosing information about FGM may place her at increased risk of harm.*

---

2 Quote from interviews conducted as part of FORWARD (2009) *FGM is Always with Us: Experiences, perceptions and beliefs of women affected by female genital mutilation in London: Results from a PEER Study*

■ *Develop a safety and support plan in case they are seen by someone 'hostile' at or near the department, venue or meeting place, e.g. agree another reason why they are there.*

■ *If they insist on being accompanied during the interview, e.g. by a teacher or advocate, ensure that the accompanying person understands the full implications of confidentiality, especially with regard to the person's family. For some, an interview may require an authorised accredited interpreter who speaks their dialect.*

■ *Do not assume that families from practising communities will want their girls and women to undergo FGM.'*

(HM Government, 2014a)

The healthcare professional should ensure that sufficient information is obtained in order to make an accurate risk assessment regarding the urgency of the situation if the individual is at risk of the procedure. The urgency may be emergency, urgent or routine. Documentation should be comprehensive and reflect the clinicians' decision-making process.

The healthcare professional must strive to establish a good rapport with their patient. This relies on using simple, comprehensible language appropriate to the patient and avoiding medical jargon, as well as on non-verbal forms of communication, such as maintaining eye contact and not being distracted by typing, telephone calls or form filling, for example.

Avoiding medical jargon, using simple language and asking straight forward questions is vital:

■ 'Have you been closed?'

■ 'Have you been opened?'

■ 'Were you circumcised?'

■ 'Have you been cut?'

Direct questions may be preferable to indirect questions, as the latter may lead to confusion and compound the patient's embarrassment.

In order to clarify the possible presence of complications, healthcare professionals should pose more direct questions, such as:

■ 'Do you experience any pains or difficulties during intercourse?'

■ 'Do you have any problems passing urine?'

■ 'Do you have difficulty passing urine?'

- 'Do you have any painful periods or pelvic pain?'
- 'Have you experienced difficulties during childbirth?'

It is important to establish a good rapport with patients so that they feel they can return to explore the issue with you in the future.

Ensure that you explain clearly and in a non-accusatory tone that FGM is illegal and that the law can help families prevent FGM being carried out on their daughters. Furthermore, highlight the potential health complications of the procedure.

Offer support such as counselling, and give information about NHS FGM specialist clinics and the government's *Statement Opposing Female Genital Mutilation* leaflet (HM Government, 2014b).

Ensure that actions taken comply with statutory and professional duties with regards to safeguarding and are in accordance with local processes and pathways.

There a number of potential barriers to patients disclosing abuse and to health professionals recognising abuse when they encounter it. Boxes 3.1 and 3.2 offer a concise summary of the main barriers to be aware of. Box 3.3 offers a summary of consultation skills that are vital when a disclosure is made.

Box 3.1: Barriers to patients disclosing abuse

- Feelings of isolation, with no-one trusted to turn to.
- The perpetrator may manipulate the patient to compound fears and anxieties that they might retaliate against the victim for disclosing, including honour-based violence.
- FGM is perceived to be an 'act of love', a once-in-a-lifetime event, and a form of abuse carried out by an otherwise loving family. Patients may therefore fear the repercussions for themselves and those close to them – fears of being taken into care and parents or loved ones being prosecuted and jailed.
- Fears of being ostracised by the community, damaging the family's honour, being unmarriageable.
- Fear of not being believed.
- Worries regarding immigration status and the possible repercussions of reporting abuse to authorities.
- Not knowing that FGM has been carried out.
- Not knowing that FGM is abuse and against the law.
- Not knowing how to vocalise the abuse due to developmental barriers and/or language barriers.

- Talking about genitalia and certain 'private' symptoms e.g. menstrual problems and lack of libido may be considered taboo.
- Lack of recognition of abuse by others, and professionals not picking up the cues.
- Anxiety over confidentiality and revelation of patient's identity.
- Lack of awareness regarding the association between FGM and the physical and psychological complications.

Box 3.2: Barriers to health professionals recognising abuse and effective safeguarding

- Not looking – abuse not being considered in the differential diagnoses.
- The rule of optimism – health professionals wanting to believe that abuse has not been carried out or is not planned.
- Not hearing the voice of the patient.
- The abuse is hidden/not obvious. The clinician needs to join the dots between the complications and FGM as the root cause.
- Lack of professional curiosity.
- Lack of multi-agency working.
- Professionals not sharing concerns appropriately.
- Professionals not owning safeguarding concerns.
- Concerns about breaking the trust and damaging the relationship between the healthcare professional and the patient/their family/their community.
- Fear of being wrong.
- Lack of confidence, knowledge and skills in how to manage the abuse and the process to follow.
- Lack of time.
- Lack of resources to support and care for patients at risk of, or survivors of, FGM.

Box 3.3: Consultation skills when a disclosure is made

- Ensure that you remain composed.
- Talk to the patient in a quiet environment, where there are no physical barriers between you and them.
- Avoid medical jargon and take care with terminology – refer to being cut/opened/closed rather than to 'female genital mutilation'.
- Ensure that you listen and support the patient, empathising with them and acknowledging their bravery in making a disclosure.
- Encourage the patient to use their own words and take their time to clarify.

- Reassure the patient that it is right to make a disclosure and they are not to blame.

- Ensure that you clarify what the patient has said and that you have understood by repeating what the patient has said and paraphrasing.

- Ensure that you have undertaken a thorough risk assessment with reference to the DoH risk assessment tool (see Box 3.5) in order to evaluate any immediate risk.

- Consider the patient's concerns regarding confidentiality and information sharing.

Ensure that your record the consultation accurately

Include the following:

- The date and time of the disclosure.

- Quote the patient's description in their own words.

- The patient's responses to what you have discussed, both verbal and non-verbal where relevant e.g. crying, agitation.

- Your plan and the justification for decisions taken.

- Your explanation to the patient of the plan, and that you will endeavour to keep them informed.

Avoid:

- Making promises you cannot keep, including undertaking to keep the abuse a secret.

- It is not your role to start/undertake the investigation.

- Do not confront an alleged perpetrator and avoid being judgemental.

- Do not be fearful of saying the wrong thing.

The 4Cs risk assessment tool

The 4Cs risk assessment tool facilitates an initial means of assessing the risk of FGM.

The tool can be used by clinicians where FGM and/or a risk of FGM is suspected. The Department of Health risk assessment tool (see Box 3.5) is a more detailed means of assessing the risk of FGM being carried out.

Box 3.4: The 4Cs

1. Do you come from a community that practices **C**utting?
2. Have you or any member of your family been **C**ut?
3. For women and girls, ask 'does anyone intend to **C**ut you or anyone you know?'
4. For patients who are pregnant or mothers of daughters ask, 'do you or anyone you know intend to have your daughter(s) **C**ut?'

A yes to at least one of these questions increases the risk of FGM and local safeguarding procedures should be followed.

© Dr Sharon Raymond

The Department of Health has recently issued a more detailed risk assessment tool and guidance regarding FGM and safeguarding, in the form of the following document: *Female Genital Mutilation Risk and Safeguarding: Guidance for professionals* (DoH, 2015a).

Using any form of guidance does not replace the need for professional judgement in relation to the circumstances presented.

Box 3.5: Safeguarding risk assessment guidance

The following information is taken from *Female Genital Mutilation Risk and Safeguarding* (DoH, 2015a). Healthcare professionals should seek to undertake an initial risk assessment, followed by the on-going assessment of girls and women.

Introductory questions

1. Do you or your partner come from a community where cutting or circumcision is practised? Remember this may relate to either one of the patient's parents' community or country of origin;
2. Have you been cut?

A YES to either of these questions would require completion of the risk template.

Part one: For an adult woman (18 years or over)

A. PREGNANT WOMAN – ask the introductory questions.

If the answer is YES to either question, use part 1(a) to support your discussions.

B. NON-PREGNANT WOMAN where you suspect FGM.

For example if a woman presents with physical symptoms or emotional behaviour that triggers a concern (e.g. frequent urinary tract infections, severe menstrual pain, infertility, symptoms of PTSD such as depression, anxiety, flashbacks or reluctance to have genital examination etc; or if FGM is discovered through the standard delivery of healthcare (e.g. when placing a urinary catheter, carrying out a smear test etc), ask the introduction questions.

If the answer is YES to either question, use part 1(b) to support your discussions.

Part two: For a CHILD (under 18 years)

Ask the introductory questions (see above) to either the child directly or the parent or legal guardian depending upon the situation.

If the answer to either question is yes OR you suspect that the child might be at risk of FGM, use part 2 to support your discussions.

Part three: For a CHILD (under 18 years)

Ask the introductory questions (see above) to either the child directly or the parent or legal guardian depending upon the situation.

If the answer to either question is yes OR you suspect that the child has had FGM, use part 3 to support your discussions.

In all circumstances:

- The woman and family must be informed of the law in the UK and the health consequences of practising FGM.

- Ensure all discussions are approached with due sensitivity and are non-judgemental.

- Any action must meet all statutory and professionals' responsibilities in relation to safeguarding, and be in line with local processes and arrangements.

- Using this guidance does not replace the need for professional judgement in relation to the circumstances presented.

Part one (a): Pregnant women

This is to help you make a decision as to whether the unborn child (or other female children in the family) are at risk of FGM or whether the woman herself is at risk of further harm in relation to her FGM.

Consider risk	yes	no	details
■ Woman comes from a community known to practice FGM			
■ Woman has undergone FGM herself			
■ Husband/partner comes from a community known to practice FGM			
■ A female family elder is involved/will be involved in care of children/unborn child or is influential in the family			
■ Woman/family has limited integration in UK community			

Consider risk	yes	no	details
■ Woman and/or husband/partner have limited/ no understanding of harm of FGM or UK law			
■ Woman's nieces of siblings and/or in-laws have undergone FGM			
■ Woman has failed to attend follow-up appointment with an FGM clinic/FGM related appointment			
■ Woman's husband/partner/other family member are very dominant in the family and have not been present during consultations with the woman			
■ Woman is reluctant to undergo genital examination			

Significant or immediate risk	yes	no	details
■ Woman already has daughters that have undergone FGM			
■ Woman is requesting reinfibulation following childbirth			
■ Woman is considered to be a vulnerable adult and therefore issues of mental capacity and consent should be considered if she is found to have FGM			
■ Woman says that FGM is integral to cultural or religious identity			
■ Family are already known to social care services – if known, and you have identified FGM within a family, you must share this information with social services			

Please remember: any child under 18 who has undergone FGM should be referred to social services.

For more information, see Action.

Part one (b): Non-pregnant adult woman (over 18)

This is to help decide whether any female children are at risk of FGM, whether there are other children in the family for whom a risk assessment may be required or whether the woman herself is at risk of further harm in relation to her FGM.

Consider risk	yes	no	details
■ Woman already has daughters who have undergone FGM – who are over 18 years of age			
■ Husband/partner comes from a community known to practice FGM			
■ Grandmother (maternal or paternal) is influential in family or female family elder is involved in care of children			
■ Woman and family have limited integration in UK community			
■ Woman's husband/partner/other family member may be very dominant in the family and have not been present during consultations with the woman			
■ Woman/family have limited/no understanding of harm of FGM or UK law			
■ Woman's nieces (by sibling or in-laws) have undergone FGM. Please note – if they are under 18 years you have a professional duty of care to refer to social care			
■ Woman has failed to attend follow-up appointment with an FGM clinic/FGM related appointment			
■ Family are already known to social services – if known, and you have identified FGM within a family, you must share this information with social services			

Significant or immediate risk	yes	no	details
■ Woman/family believe FGM is integral to cultural or religious identity			
■ Woman already has daughters who have undergone FGM – who are under 18 years of age			
■ Woman is considered to be a vulnerable adult and therefore issues of mental capacity and consent should be considered if she is has had FGM			

Any child under 18 who has undergone FGM should be referred to social services.

Part two: Child/young adult (under 18 years old)

This is to help when considering whether a child is AT RISK of FGM, or whether there are other children in the family for whom a risk assessment may be required.

Consider risk	yes	no	details
■ Child's mother has undergone FGM			
■ Other female family members have had FGM			
■ Father comes from a community known to practice FGM			
■ A family elder such as Grandmother is very influential within the family and is/will be involved in the care of the girl			
■ Mother/family have limited contact with people outside of her family			
■ Parents have poor access to information about FGM and do not know about the harmful effects of FGM or UK law			
■ Parents say that they or a relative will be taking the girl abroad for a prolonged period – this may not only be to a country with high prevalence, but this would more likely lead to a concern			
■ Girl has spoken about a long holiday to her country of origin/another country where the practice is prevalent			
■ Girl has attended a travel clinic or equivalent for vaccinations/anti-malarials			
■ FGM is referred to in conversation by the child, family or close friends of the child – the context of the discussion will be important			
■ Sections missing from the Red book. Consider if the child has received immunisations, do they attend clinics etc			
■ Girl withdrawn from PHSE lessons or from learning about FGM – school nurse should have conversation with child			
■ Girls presents symptoms that could be related to FGM – continue with questions in part 3			
■ Family not engaging with professionals (health, school, or other)			

Significant or immediate risk	yes	no	details
■ A child or sibling asks for help			
■ A parent or family member expresses concern that FGM may be carried out on the child			
■ Girl has confided in another that she is to have a 'special procedure' or to attend a 'special occasion'. Girl has talked about going away 'to become a woman' or 'to become like my mum and sister'			
■ Girl has a sister or other female child relative who has already undergone FGM			
■ Family/child are already known to social services – if known, and you have identified FGM within a family, you must share this information with social services			

Please remember: any child under 18 who has undergone FGM should be referred to social services.

Part three: Child/young adult (under 18 years old)

This is to help when considering whether a child HAS HAD FGM.

Consider risk	yes	no	details
■ Girl is reluctant to undergo any medical examination			
■ Girl has difficulty walking, sitting or standing or looks uncomfortable			
■ Girl finds it hard to sit still for long periods of time, which was not a problem previously			
■ Girl presents to GP or A&E with frequent urine, menstrual or stomach problems			
■ Increased emotional and psychological needs e.g. withdrawal, depression, or significant change in behaviour			
■ Girl avoiding physical exercise or requiring to be excused from PE lessons without a GP's letter			
■ Girl has spoken about having been on a long holiday to her country of origin/ another country where the practice is prevalent			

Consider risk	yes	no	details
■ Girl spends a long time in the bathroom/toilet/long periods of time away from the classroom ■ Girl talks about pain or discomfort between her legs			

Significant or immediate risk	yes	no	details
■ Girl asks for help ■ Girl confides in a professional that FGM has taken place ■ Mother/family member discloses that female child has had FGM ■ Family/child are already known to social services – if known, and you have identified FGM within a family, you must share this information with social services			

Please remember: any child under 18 who has undergone FGM should be referred to social services.

Action

- ■ Ask more questions – if one indicator leads to a potential area of concern, continue the discussion in this area.

- ■ Consider risk – if one or more indicators are identified, you need to consider what action to take. If unsure whether the level of risk requires referral at this point, discuss with your named/designated safeguarding lead.

- ■ Significant or immediate risk – if you identify one or more serious or immediate risk, or the other risks are, by your judgement, sufficient to be considered serious, you should look to refer to Social Services/CAIT team/Police/MASH, in accordance with your local safeguarding procedures.

If the risk of harm is imminent, emergency measures may be required and any action taken must reflect the required urgency.

In all cases:

- ■ Share information of any identified risk with the patient's GP
- ■ Document in notes
- ■ Discuss the health complications of FGM and the law in the UK

(DoH, 2015a © Crown copyright 2015. Contains public sector information lisensed under the Open Government Licence v3.0. To view this licence, visit www.nationalarchives.gov.uk/doc/open-government.licence/)

Management of FGM

When managing a patient who may have undergone FGM, ensure that you manage the physical and psychological complications of FGM and that appropriate referrals are made. This may include referral to secondary care for physical complications in relation to, for example, menstrual problems and recurrent urinary tract infections.

Many women who have undergone type 3 FGM should be offered the procedure known as 'deinfibulation'. This minor surgical procedure entails the opening of the vaginal opening under local anaesthetic, and is usually undertaken as an outpatient. It may entail referral to an FGM specialist clinic.

Under certain circumstances, deinfibulation may be undertaken under general anaesthetic, such as where there is significant local scarring, where there are clitoral cysts, or where there are marked psychological complications e.g. PTSD. Should the patient be pregnant, a spinal anaesthetic is preferred to a general anaesthetic.

Deinfibulation may in particular be indicated in women who are of child bearing age or are pregnant, as failure to undertake the procedure may place both mother and baby at serious risk. For women who are pregnant, deinfibulation is best undertaken during the second trimester. Patients may prefer to undergo the deinfibulation procedure during labour, and this should be clearly documented in her notes.

Regarding psychological support, a referral to the local mental health team or to an FGM clinic offering psychological support may be indicated.

FGM is often undertaken due to a range of complex motives and patients' and their families' needs may best be clarified with the involvement of interpreters and health advocates. An accredited female interpreter may be required. Any interpreter should ideally be appropriately trained in relation to FGM and in all cases should not be a family member, not be known to the individual, and not be an individual with any standing or power within the patient's community, as patients may feel embarrassed to broach sensitive and personal matters in their presence and be fearful that this information may be transmitted to other members of their community, thereby placing the patient in danger.

Furthermore, interpreters from the patient's family or their community may purposefully mislead clinicians, or pressurise the patient not to pursue a complaint and to succumb to the wishes of their family and community.

It is also important to signpost patients and their families to the third sector and community groups where appropriate as sources of additional support, such as Southall Black Sisters or the NSPCC Helpline, which professionals should be aware of. This helpline can support both professionals or family members concerned that a child is at risk of, or has had FGM.

Two important points that bear repeating when managing a patient who may have undergone FGM or who may be at risk of this practice are as follows:

1. Ensure you have fulfilled your professional safeguarding duties in line your duty of care, in accordance with current national and local guidance.

2. Inform patients about the illegality of FGM, which is a clear abuse of women and children, and outline the potential complications of FGM, highlighting the possible harm that this procedure can cause.

Safeguarding children and young and vulnerable adults

While specific legislation and guidance is in place regarding FGM, healthcare professionals must also be guided by all existing safeguarding adults and children legislation, both international and national, as well as professional guidance including The Care Act (2014), The Mental Capacity Act (2005) and (2010), The Human Rights Act (1998), The UN Convention on the Rights of the Child (1989), the Children Acts (1989 and 2004) (for England and Wales), and the Children (Northern Ireland) Order (1995).

The Department for Education published an updated version of the key statutory guidance for anyone working with children in England in March 2015, titled *Working Together to Safeguard Children* (HM Government, 2015) in England. This document guides professionals in working together in the assessment and safeguarding of children, updating the 2013 version.

It is the healthcare professional's duty to ensure that children and vulnerable adults are safeguarded from FGM. It is important to note that as with other forms of abuse against adults, healthcare professionals are not required to refer women automatically who they do not deem to be vulnerable adults to the police or social care.

When a professional discovers a case of FGM in an adult or child, it is important to establish where and when it took place when establishing the potential risk to other individuals. In the case of adult patients who are not deemed to be vulnerable, healthcare professionals need to assess whether there is an indication to report a case of FGM or the risk of FGM if there may be risk to others, including any children or vulnerable adults, and/or if there is a public interest to do so.

Box 3.6: FGM and forced marriage

An association has been established between those individuals experiencing FGM and forced marriage. Healthcare professionals should follow best practice guidance in safeguarding patients at risk. The multi-agency practice guidelines on the management of cases of forced marriages can be found at: https://www.gov.uk/forced-marriage#guidance-for-professionals.

FGM is child abuse and Section 47 of the Children Act (1989) stipulates that anyone who has information that a child is potentially or actually at risk of significant harm must inform social care or the police. Professionals must always ensure that they inform social services or the police.

If a child or young woman under 18 years of age is suspected by a healthcare professional to have undergone FGM or be at risk of this practice, a referral must be made to social care in accordance with safeguarding procedures in place for all forms of child abuse and suspected abuse. In the in-hours setting this should usually be to the MASH i.e. the Multi-Agency Safeguarding Hub (in areas that have one), however, safeguarding referral pathways will depend on referral pathways in place locally. In the out-of-hours setting, referral should be to the duty social worker.

The new mandatory reporting duty introduced by the Serious Crime Act (2015), which will likely come into force towards the end of 2015, requires reporting of FGM in under 18 year olds to the police, and the process for this awaits clarification but is likely to be via the MASH (again, in areas that have one).

Strategic bodies should ensure that their member agencies operate effectively following policies and procedures that have been put in place to manage FGM.

Safeguarding plans are determined by multi-agency assessments (such as the Common Assessment Framework in England and the Framework for the Assessment of Children in Need and their Families in Wales).

Box 3.7: A note on making enquiries

The *Multi-Agency Practice Guidelines: Female genital mutilation* contains the following advice:

'In general, enquiries should be undertaken by police officers with assistance from social workers. However, there may be occasions when professionals may wish to make informal enquiries before involving police if, for example, a girl has been absent from school for a prolonged period. In these circumstances, it is important not to reveal that enquiries are related to FGM as this may increase the risk to the girl or woman. If the fact that the enquiries relate to FGM needs to be shared, this should only be shared with professionals aware of the need to handle such information appropriately.'

(HM Government, 2014a)

Information sharing, consent and confidentiality

The *Multi-Agency Practice Guidelines* (HM Government, 2014a) advise as follows:

'To safeguard children and young people as required by UK law, it may be necessary to give information to people working in other agencies or departments.

For some professionals, this can pose dilemmas when it involves going beyond the normal boundaries of confidentiality. Nonetheless, both law and policy allow for disclosure where it is in the public interest or where a criminal act may have been perpetrated. There may also be the perception that passing on information can damage the relationship of trust built up with families and communities. However, it is crucial that the focus is kept on the best interests of the child as required by law.

Guidance about disclosure and when confidentiality can be breached is available in the following publications:

- ■ *What to Do if You are Worried a Child is Being Abused (HM Government, 2015). https://www.gov.uk/government/uploads/system/uploads/attachment_data/file/419604/What_to_do_if_you_re_worried_a_child_is_being_abused.pdf*
- ■ *Nursing and Midwifery Council's Advice on confidentiality (2009).*
- ■ *General Medical Council's guidance (2009) Confidentiality. See http://www.gmc-uk.org/Confidentiality___English_0415.pdf_48902982.pdf*

■ *Guidance on the Management of Police Information. See http://www. app.college.police.uk/*

Referrals to other professionals or agencies should be conducted using existing and agreed procedures and arrangements. However, there may be times when a victim wants to take a course of action that may put them at risk – on these occasions, professionals should explain all the outcomes and risks to the victim and take the necessary child or adult protection precautions. Professionals should also be clear that FGM is a criminal offence in the UK and must not be permitted or condoned.'

(HM Government, 2014 © Crown copyright)

Working Together to Safeguard Children (HM Government, 2015) lays out guidance on information sharing for healthcare professionals, which can often be a challenging area for clinicians.

The document highlights the crucial importance of the effective sharing of information between professionals and local agencies in order to best identify, assess and provide the right services.

Healthcare professionals should strive to share information in a timely manner in order to facilitate help at the earliest possible opportunity where there are evolving problems. Sharing information is of key importance in ensuring child protection services are initiated without unnecessary delay. A recurrent theme in serious case reviews (SCRs) is a lack of effective information sharing between agencies, culminating in child deaths and abuse of children.

Healthcare professionals should not allow concerns regarding information sharing to delay or interfere with safeguarding duties, always ensuring that the welfare of the child is paramount.

Effective safeguarding depends on the following:

■ Agencies should ensure that systems are in place specifying the principles and processes of information sharing between professionals and agencies.

■ Healthcare professionals should take care not to assume that another professional has shared information necessary to safeguarding a child or adult in a vulnerable situation. It is every professionals' duty to own and share their concerns with social care where there is a risk that a child or adult in a vulnerable situation has suffered or may suffer harm.

Information Sharing: Guidance for practitioners providing safeguarding services to children, young people, parents and carers (DfE, 2015) provides guidance in best practice for professionals required to make decisions about the sharing of information, including the seven golden rules for effective information sharing.

Regarding adults with capacity, as distinct from adults in a vulnerable situation, it is acknowledged that they have the capacity to make decisions in their own interests, including what professionals may deem to be unwise decisions, such as whether or not they consent to sharing confidential information. If a woman does decline to consent to sharing information, and this does into put other individuals at risk, it ought to be respected, but healthcare professionals need to support patients when making decisions regarding the disclosure of personal information and encourage them to share information with services that may help them cope with the complications of FGM.

Healthcare professionals should also undertake a risk assessment and evaluate whether there may be a public interest in breaching a patient's confidentiality without their consent, including if this would aid in preventing, detecting or prosecuting a crime, or if not sharing information may place another individual at risk of harm.

FGM risk indication system

As of summer 2015, there will be a system available via the NHS Summary Care Record application that facilitates the recording on a child's healthcare record that she may be at risk of FGM during her lifetime. This information will act as a prompt for healthcare professionals to evaluate the risk of FGM when they deliver care in the future.

The efficacy of the FGM risk indication system relies on healthcare professionals' having the appropriate level of knowledge and skills regarding the evaluation of the risk of FGM. The risk assessment tool in Box 3.5 (p48) serves as a tool to guide the ongoing monitoring and review of the risk of FGM.

At the time of going to print, further information regarding this system is awaited.

Box 3.8: GMC guidance relating to doctors dealing with cases of FGM

As well as the *Multi-Agency Practice Guidelines: FGM* (HM Government, 2014a), which provides guidance for each agency involved in caring and safeguarding women and girls who have undergone or are at risk of FGM, specific guidance exists for some of the key healthcare professional groups. Nurses and midwives can refer to *Female Genital Mutilation: An RCN resource for nursing and midwifery practice* (RCN, 2015), and there is also guidance issued by the Royal College of Obstetricians and Gynaecologists in 2015.

The GMC offers the following guidance:

- 'You must be familiar with guidelines and developments that affect your work.'[1]

- 'You must keep up-to-date with, and follow, the law, our guidance and other regulations relevant to your work.'[2]

- 'Under child protection guidance FGM is a safeguarding issue. You must report concerns that a child has suffered, or may be at risk of serious harm to an appropriate agency – such as the police, local authority children's service or NSPCC – unless there are exceptional reasons for believing it would not be in the best interests of the child to do so. This applies to concerns about FGM.'[3]

- 'You do not need to be certain that the child or young person is at risk of significant harm to take this step. If a child or young person is at risk of, or is suffering, abuse or neglect the potential consequences of not sharing relevant information will, in the vast majority of cases, outweigh any harm that sharing your concerns with an appropriate agency might cause.'[4]

- 'You should develop an understanding of the practices and beliefs of the different cultural and religious communities you serve.'[5]

- 'In the case of adults, if a woman refuses consent for information to be shared, and that decision does not leave anyone else at risk of harm, GMC guidance advises that her decision should usually be respected.[6] Therefore, you should consult with the woman, about ways in which to proceed and should focus on supporting and empowering the woman to make decisions about disclosure of information about her. You should also encourage the woman to contact, or agree to disclosure to, services that can support her in dealing with the impact of FGM on her.'

- 'There can, however, be a public interest justification for sharing information about a woman without her consent if doing so would assist in the prevention, detection or prosecution of serious crime or if failure to do so would leave others at risk of harm.'[7]

1 GMC (2013), paragraph 11   2 GMC (2013), paragraph 12   3 GMC (2012)   4 GMC (2012)
5 GMC (2009), paragraph 9   6 GMC (2009), paragraph 51   7 GMC (2009), paragraph 54

Scenarios

The following six scenarios explore some of the challenges of managing FGM in clinical practice.

What are your concerns and what do you do in each of these case scenarios? In order to guide your approach to management consider the following:

- the probability of FGM, bearing in mind patients' ethnic origin – remember patients and/or their partners or families may be of mixed ethnicity.
- the possible physical and psychological complications of FGM and how to manage these, including supporting survivors in coping with the consequences of FGM, and referral to secondary care and deinfibulation clinics where indicated.
- Any risk to your patients and other females in line with healthcare professionals' safeguarding duties, including the duty to consider the public interest.

Case scenario 1

A 20-year-old Egyptian woman comes to see you complaining of a three-day-history of dysuria. She has been suffering with recurrent urinary tract infections for the last 10 years.

- She appears anxious.
- She came to the UK with her family eight years ago and lives with her parents and two younger sisters.
- She discloses that she was cut at the age of nine years.

Case scenario 2

- A 40-year-old mother of five, originally from Somalia, comes to see her GP about a flare up of her eczema.
- As you examine her skin she mentions that life at home is becoming increasingly difficult due to regular arguments with her husband.
- They don't seem to agree on much lately and her husband wants to arrange a family trip to Somalia over the summer to visit relatives and friends. She is withdrawn and her mood appears low.

Case scenario 3

A school nurse is concerned regarding an 11-year-old female pupil who has recently returned from a family trip to Ethiopia. She is spending long periods in the toilet and seems in some discomfort walking and sitting in class.

Case scenario 4

A practice nurse is concerned regarding a young Nigerian woman she has just seen. She is three months pregnant but has not yet attended the surgery as she says she fears being examined and giving birth. Her sister's labour lasted for three days, in which both her and her child nearly died.

Case scenario 5

A father comes to see the practice nurse with his five children for travel vaccinations prior to a trip to Egypt. Two of the children are girls aged nine and 14 years who have never been to Egypt in the past. The nine-year-old discloses to the nurse that she is looking forward to a big ceremony Dad has organised, and mum has been buying her dresses and gifts in preparation for this coming-of-age party.

Case scenario 6

A 60-year-old Dutch widower presents with what appears to be PTSD – she has been having flashbacks of a traumatic event she experienced some 20 years ago. She has no children and lives alone. During the course of the consultation you discover that 20 years ago she was in a brief relationship with a partner from a practising community who insisted that she undergo FGM.

Conclusion: the challenges posed by FGM

In order to ensure best practice in caring for patients who are at risk of or who have undergone FGM, healthcare professionals working within their multi-agency teams must strive to ensure that they have undertaken the appropriate training in accordance with professional training guidelines. The intercollegiate guidelines *Safeguarding Children and Young People: Roles and competencies for healthcare staff* (RCPCH, 2014) highlight FGM as a mandatory competency for safeguarding children training. Furthermore, professionals must ensure that they are aware of and follow national and local guidelines and processes in managing FGM.

Healthcare professionals must ensure that they fulfil their duty of care to patients by managing the complications of FGM and safeguarding children and vulnerable adults at risk of FGM in accordance with statutory safeguarding guidance and best practice guidelines, and communicate with patients sensitively, highlighting the fact that FGM is against the law and the complications that it can lead to.

Healthcare professionals working within their multi-agency teams should aim to establish a robust approach to undertaking the ongoing risk assessment of children and young women, where the initial risk of FGM being performed has been deemed to be low.

FGM services are in place across the UK, though as highlighted by *Commissioning Services to Support Women and Girls with Female Genital Mutilation* (DoH, 2015b), the commissioning of FGM services will need to be developed in response to local needs as evidenced by increasingly more robust national prevalence data.

The development of FGM specialist clinics across the country has tended to be prompted by local healthcare professionals and FGM campaigners observing a need for these services and taking the initiative.

The collation of statistics on FGM will help guide commissioners in building a national picture of patient needs, facilitating greater central direction in establishing FGM services where they are required.

There remains a need for additional central guidance regarding healthcare professionals' approach to and management of genital piercing, which is deemed to be FGM by the legislation, and female genital cosmetic surgery, which may in some cases be considered to be FGM. Furthermore, healthcare professionals await clear guidance regarding the processes for the mandatory reporting of FGM in under 18 year olds in accordance with the Serious Crime Act (2015). Guidance is in the process of being delivered, as are the necessary services to be tailored to patients' needs.

Best practice in the management of FGM relies on well-trained professionals working together in accordance with national and local policies and processes, and the presence of sufficient resources to ensure that women and girls receive the care that they need and deserve to help prevent or better cope with FGM – a hidden scar, the effects of which can be potentially devastating and life-long.

References

Department for Education (2015) *Information Sharing: Guidance for practitioners providing safeguarding services to children, young people, parents and carers* [online]. Available at: https://www.gov.uk/government/publications/safeguarding-practitioners-information-sharing-advice (accessed August 2015).

Department of Health (2015a) *Female Genital Mutilation Risk and Safeguarding: Guidance for professionals* [online]. London: DoH. Available at: https://www.gov.uk/government/uploads/system/uploads/attachment_data/file/418564/2903800_DH_FGM_Accessible_v0.1.pdf (accessed August 2015).

Department of Health (2015b) *Commissioning Services to Support Women and Girls with Female Genital Mutilation* [online]. Available at: https://www.gov.uk/government/uploads/system/uploads/attachment_data/file/418549/2903842_DH_FGM_Commissioning_Accessible.pdf (accessed August 2015).

GMC (2009) *Confidentiality* [online]. London: General Medical Council. Available at: http://www.gmc-uk.org/static/documents/content/Confidentiality_-_english.pdf (accessed August 2015).

GMC (2012) *Protecting Children and Young People: The responsibilities of all doctors* [online]. London: General Medical Council. Available at: http://www.gmc-uk.org/static/documents/content/Protecting_children_and_young_people_English_0315.pdf (accessed August 2015).

GMC (2013) *Good Medical Practice* [online]. London: General Medical Council. Available at: http://www.gmc-uk.org/static/documents/content/Good_medical_practice_-_English_0914.pdf (accessed August 2015).

HM Government (2014a) *Multi-Agency Practice Guidelines: Female genital mutilation* [online]. London: HM Government. Available at: https://www.gov.uk/government/uploads/system/uploads/attachment_data/file/380125/MultiAgencyPracticeGuidelinesNov14.pdf (accessed August 2015).

HM Government (2014b) *A Statement Opposing Female Genital Mutilation* [online]. London: HM Government. Available at: https://www.gov.uk/government/uploads/system/uploads/attachment_data/file/378132/FGMstatementNov14.pdf (accessed August 2015).

HM Government (2015) *Working Together to Safeguard Children: A guide to inter-agency working to safeguard and promote the welfare of children* [online]. London: DfE. Available at: https://www.gov.uk/government/uploads/system/uploads/attachment_data/file/419595/Working_Together_to_Safeguard_Children.pdf (accessed August 2015).

Royal College of Paediatrics and Child Health (2014) *Safeguarding Children and Young People: Roles and competencies for healthcare staff* [online]. Available at: http://www.apagbi.org.uk/sites/default/files/images/Safeguarding%20Children%20-%20Roles%20andCompetences%20for%20Healthcare%20Staff%20%2002%200....pdf (accessed August 2015).

Royal College of Nursing (2015) *Female Genital Mutilation: An RCN resource for nursing and midwifery practice* [online]. Available at: http://www.rcn.org.uk/__data/assets/pdf_file/0010/608914/RCNguidance_FGM_WEB2.pdf (accessed August 2015).

Royal College of Obstetricians and Gynaecologists (2015) *Female Genital Mutilation and Its Management* [online]. Available at: www.rcog.org.uk/en/guidelines-research-services/guidelines/gtg53/ (accessed August 2015).

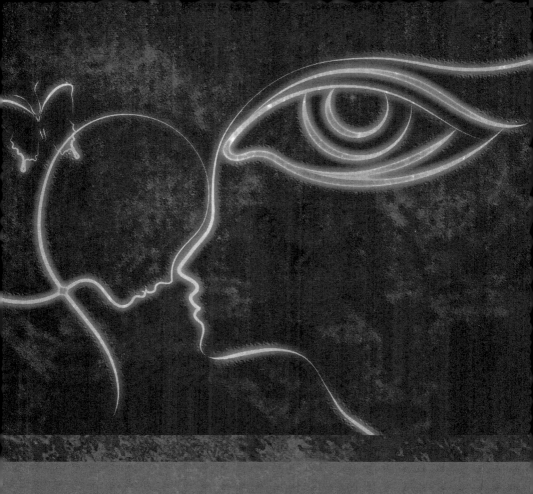

Further resources

Further resources

The NHS currently offers free e-learning training about FGM to all health professionals. For more information, visit http://www.e-lfh.org.uk/programmes/female-genital-mutilation.

For further support materials and videos including patient information leaflets and health passports in 11 languages, visit www.nhs.uk/fgmguidelines

NHS specialist services for FGM

London

African Women's Clinic: University College London Hospitals NHS Foundation Trust

Address:
Elizabeth Garrett Anderson Wing
University College London
Lower Ground Floor
25 Grafton Way
London
WC1E 6DB

e-mail: For complex cases, sohier.elneil@uclh.nhs.uk or fgmsupport@uclh.nhs.uk
Telephone: 07944 241992

For more information, see http://www.uclh.nhs.uk/OurServices/OurHospitals/UCH/EGAWing/Pages/Home.aspx

Acton African Well Woman Clinic: Imperial College Healthcare NHS Trust

Address:
Acton Health Centre 35
61 Church Road
London
W3 8QE

Telephone: 07956 001 065 or 0208 383 8761 or 07730970738

Queen Charlotte's & Chelsea Hospital African Well Woman Clinic: Imperial College Healthcare NHS Trust

Address:
Du Cane Road
London
W12 0HS

Telephone: 07956 001 065 or 0208 383 8761 or 07730970738

West London African Women's Service: Chelsea and Westminster Hospital NHS Trust

Sexual health:
West London Centre for Sexual Health

Address:
West London Centre for Sexual Health
Charing Cross Hospital (South Wing)
Fulham Palace Road
London
W6 8RF

Telephone: 0208 846 1579 (Health Advisors)
Fax: 0203 311 7582

Maternity/gynaecology:
Chelsea and Westminster Hospital & West London Centre for Sexual Health

Address:
Chelsea and Westminster Hospital
369 Fulham Road
London
SW10 9NH

Telephone: 020 3315 3344 (Debora Alcayde, Specialist FGM Midwife)

Email enquires (all aspects of the service): caw-tr.fgmwestlondon@nhs.net

St Marys Hospital: Imperial College Healthcare NHS Trust – Well Women Clinic

Address:
Well Women Clinic
Gynaecology & Midwifery Department
Praed St.
London
W2 1NY

Telephone: 0207 886 6691 or 0207 886 1443. Helpline: 0203 312 6135

African Well Women's Clinic: Whittington Hospital

Address:
African Well Women's Clinic
Kenwood Wing
Antenatal Clinic
Level 5
Highgate Hill
London
N19 5NF

Telephone: 0207 2883482/3 or 07956257992 to make or change an appointment.

African Well Women's Clinic: Guys & St Thomas' Hospital
Address:
Guy's & St. Thomas's Hospital
African Well Women's Clinic
8th Floor – c/o Antenatal Clinic
Lambeth Palace Rd
London
SE1 7EH

Telephone: 0207 188 6872

Mile End Hospital: Barts Health NHS Trust

Address:
Women's and Young People's Services
Sylvia Pankhurst Health Centre, 3rd Floor
Bancroft road
London
E1 4DG

Telephone: 0207 377 7898 or 0207 377 7870 0208 223 8322

For more information, see: www.bartsandthelondon.nhs.uk

Northwick Park Hospital & Central Middlesex Hospital: African Well Women's Clinic – North West London Hospitals NHS Trust

Address:
African Well Women's Clinic, Antenatal Clinic
Watford road
Harrow
Middlesex
HA1 3UJ

Telephone:
Central Middlesex Hospital Park Royal Antenatal clinic 020 8453 2108
Northwick Park Hospital Harrow Antenatal clinic 020 8869 2880
nwlh-tr.PALS@nhs.net

For more information, see: http://www.nwlh.nhs.uk/services/antenatal-care/

Nottingham

Nottingham University Hospital: Nottingham University Hospitals NHS Trust – City Hospital Campus

Address:
Antenatal Clinic, Nottingham City Hospital
Hucknall Road
Nottingham
NG5 1PB

Telephone: 0115 969 1169

Bristol

Minority Ethnic Women's & Girl's Clinic: Bristol Charlotte Keel Centre

Address:
Charlotte Keel Health Centre
Seymour Road
Easton
Bristol
BS5 0UA

Telephone:
0117 9027138
0117 902 7111 (direct line)
0117 902 7100 (switchboard)
mgw@gp-L81092.nhs.uk

For more information, see: www.eastonfamilypractice.co.uk

Bristol Community Rose Clinic: Lawrence Hill Health Centre

Address:
Hassell Drive
Lawrence Hill
Bristol
BS2 0AN

Telephone: Contact Dr Katrina Darke at Lawrence Hill Heath Centre on: 07813016911or talk to your GP regarding a referral.
Email: bristolroseclinic@nhs.net

For more information, see: http://www.bristolccg.nhs.uk/media/32270/bcrclinic_mulitilingual.pdf

Birmingham

Birmingham Heartlands Hospital: Heart of England NHS Foundation Trust

Address:
Princess of Wales Women's Unit
Heartlands Hospital
Bordesley Green
East Birmingham
B9 5SS

Telephone: 0121 424 3909

Liverpool

Link Clinic: Liverpool Women's Hospital

Address:
Antenatal Clinic
Crown Street
Liverpool
Merseyside
L8 7SS

Telephone: 0151 702 4180 or 0151 702 4178

For more information, see: http://www.liverpoolwomens.nhs.uk/Our_Services/Maternity/Specialist_antenatal_clinics.aspx

Organisations working on FGM-related issues

The remaining information in this section is taken from Multi-Agency *Practice Guidelines: Female genital mutilation*, which is available at www.gov.uk/government/uploads/system/uploads/attachment_data/file/380125/MultiAgencyPracticeGuidelinesNov14.pdf. © Crown copyright 2014. Contains public sector information licensed under the Open Government Licence v3.0. To view this licence, visit: www.nationalarchives.gov.uk/doc/open-government-licence/

Police service

Metropolitan Police Service / Project Azure
020 7161 2888

UK Government

https://www.gov.uk/female-genital-mutilation

Helplines

National Society for the Prevention of Cruelty to Children (NSPCC) FGM Helpline
24-hour helpline. Freephone 0800 028 3550
www.nspcc.org.uk/fgm

Black Association of Women Step Out (BAWSO)
24-hour helpline: 0800 731 8147
www.bawso.org.uk

ChildLine
24-hour helpline for children: 0800 1111
www.childline.org.uk

National Domestic Violence Helpline
24-hour helpline: 0808 2000 247
www.nationaldomesticviolencehelpline.org.uk

NSPCC British Sign Language Helpline for deaf or hard-of-hearing callers
ISDN videophone: 020 8463 1148
Webcam: nspcc.signvideo.tv (available Monday –
Friday, 9am–5pm, in English language only)
Text: 0800 056 0566

Other organisations

28 Too Many
http://28toomany.org/

Africans Unite Against Child Abuse (AFRUCA)
http://www.afruca.org/

Agency for Culture and Change Management UK (ACCM UK)
http://www.accmuk.com/

Birmingham & Solihull Women's Aid
http://bswaid.org/

Foundation for Women's Health Research & Development (FORWARD)
http://www.forwarduk.org.uk/

Halo Project
http://www.haloproject.org.uk/

Manor Gardens Health Advocacy Project
http://www.manorgardenscentre.org/

The Maya Centre
www.mayacentre.org.uk

For more organisations and local services visit https://www.gov.uk/female-genital-mutilation

FGM reference materials

Guidance and guidelines for professionals

The following list is not designed to be an exhaustive list of all applicable publications. Professionals should consult the relevant professional bodies and agencies for the up-to-date guidance.

- All Wales Child Protection Procedures Review Group (2011) *All Wales Protocol: Female genital mutilation*. Available at: http://www.awcpp. org.uk/wp-content/uploads/2014/03/Female-Genital-Mutilation.pdf (accessed August 2015)

- Association of Chief Police Officers (2009) *Guidance on Investigating Child Abuse and Safeguarding Children* (2nd Ed). Available at: https://www.ceop.police.uk/Documents/ACPOGuidance2009.pdf (Accessed August 2015)

- Department for Children, Schools and Families (2013) *Working Together to Safeguard Children: A guide to inter-agency working to safeguard and promote the welfare of children*. Available at: https:// www.gov.uk/government/uploads/system/uploads/attachment_data/ file/417669/Archived-Working_together_to_safeguard_children.pdf (accessed August 2015)

- British Medical Association (2011) *Female Genital Mutilation: Caring for patients and child protection*. London: BMA

■ General Medical Council (2012) *Raising and Acting on Concerns about Patient Safety*. Available at: http://www.gmc-uk.org/guidance/ethical_guidance/raising_concerns.asp (accessed August 2015)

■ General Medical Council (2007) *0–18 Years: Guidance for all doctors*. Available at: http://www.gmc-uk.org/guidance/ethical_guidance/children_guidance_index.asp (accessed August 2015)

■ General Medical Council (2008) *Consent: Patients and doctors making decisions together*. Available at: http://www.gmc-uk.org/guidance/ethical_guidance/consent_guidance_index.asp (accessed August 2015)

■ General Medical Council (2009) *Confidentiality*. Available at: http://www.gmc-uk.org/guidance/ethical_guidance/confidentiality.asp (accessed August 2015)

■ HM Government (2015) *What to Do if You are Worried a Child is Being Abused*. Available at: https://www.gov.uk/government/uploads/system/uploads/attachment_data/file/419604/What_to_do_if_you_re_worried_a_child_is_being_abused.pdf (accessed August 2015)

■ HM Government (2009) *Multi-Agency Practice Guidelines: Handling cases of forced marriage*. Available at: https://www.gov.uk/government/uploads/system/uploads/attachment_data/file/35530/forced-marriage-guidelines09.pdf (accessed August 2015)

■ HM Government (2012) *Call to End Violence against Women and Girls: Taking action – the next chapter*. Available at: https://www.gov.uk/government/uploads/system/uploads/attachment_data/file/97901/action-plan-new-chapter.pdf (accessed August 2015)

■ Standardisation Committee for Care Information (2014) *Female Genital Mutilation Prevalence Dataset*

■ Nursing and Midwifery Council (2008) *The Code: Standards of conduct, performance and ethics for nurses and midwives*. Available at: http://www.nmc.org.uk/globalassets/sitedocuments/standards/the-code-a4-20100406.pdf (accessed August 2015)

■ Royal College of Midwives, Royal College of Nursing, Royal College of Obstetricians and Gynaecologists, Equality Now & UNITE (2013) *Tackling FGM in the UK: Intercollegiate recommendations for identifying, recording and reporting*. Available at: http://www.equalitynow.org/sites/default/files/Intercollegiate_FGM_report.pdf (accessed August 2015)

■ Royal College of Midwives (2011) *RCM Position Statement: Female Genital Mutilation*. Further information available at: https://www.rcm.org.uk/tags/fgm (accessed August 2015)

■ Royal College of Midwives (2011) *Guidance for Midwives*

- Royal College of Nursing (2015) *Female Genital Mutilation: An RCN educational resource for nursing and midwifery staff* (2nd Ed). Available at: http://www.rcn.org.uk/__data/assets/pdf_file/0010/608914/RCNguidance_FGM_WEB2.pdf (accessed August 2015)

- Royal College of Obstetricians and Gynaecologists (2015) *Female Genital Mutilation and Its Management* [online]. Available at: www.rcog.org.uk/en/guidelines-research-services/guidelines/ gtg53/ (accessed August 2015).

- Welsh Assembly Government (2004) *Safeguarding Children: Working together to safeguard children under the Children Act 2004*. Available at: http://www.wales.nhs.uk/sitesplus/863/opendoc/204221 (accessed August 2015)

The FGM National Clinical Group has produced an educational DVD which clearly instructs and shows doctors, midwives and nurses how to undertake de-infibulation. This can be ordered from the group's website: www.fgmnationalgroup.org

An NHS Choices FGM page containing information and support for frontline professionals and members of the public who are concerned about the practice and are seeking advice is available at: www.nhs.uk/fgm.

A Department of Health DVD about FGM can be also ordered by emailing fgm@dh.gsi.gov.uk

Information about the government's strategy to eradicate violence against women and girls can be found at https://www.gov.uk/government/ policies/ ending-violence-against-women-and-girls-in-the-uk

Information from the Department for Education about safeguarding children can be found at https://www.gov.uk/childrens-services/ safeguarding-children

Government-produced leaflets and posters

Professionals, civil society partners and members of the public can request copies of the government's leaflets, posters and latest DVD about FGM from FGMEnquiries@homeoffice.gsi.gov.uk

Outreach and peer support

The government's FGM unit can offer advice and support to local areas who would like to strengthen or develop their work on tackling FGM.

To contact the FGM unit, please email: FGMEnquiries@homeoffice.gsi.gov.uk

More information on the role of the FGM unit can be found at:
https://www.gov.uk/government/collections/female-genital-mutilation

To view some examples of effective practice in tackling FGM, please visit:
https://www.gov.uk/government/publications/female-genital-mutilation-resource-pack

Books

Comfort Momoh, *Female Genital Mutilation* (ISBN 9781857756937)
Waris Dirie, *Desert Flower* (ISBN 9780688158231)
Layli Miller Bashir and Fauziya assindja, *Do They Hear You When You Cry?* (ISBN 9780553505634)
Alice Walker, *Possessing the Secret of Joy* (ISBN 9780671789428)
Tasmin Bradley, *Women, Violence and Tradition: Taking FGM and other practices to a secular state* (ISBN 9781848139589)
Susannah Carlton, *Biting The Stick* (ISBN 9781497363489)

Research about FGM

FORWARD (2007) A Statistical Study to Estimate the Prevalence of Female Genital Mutilation in England and Wales http://www.forwarduk.org.uk/key-issues/ fgm/research

(To view other FORWARD resources and publications, please visit http://www.forwarduk.org.uk/resources)

UNICEF (2013) Female Genital Mutilation/ Cutting: A statistical overview and exploration of the dynamics of change http://www.unicef.org/media/files/FGCM_Lo_ res.pdf

EIGE (2013) Female Genital Mutilation in the European Union and Croatia http://eige.europa.eu/sites/default/files/ EIGE-Report-FGM-in-the-EU-and-Croatia_0.Pdf